Frankly
PREGNANT

Frankly
PREGNANT

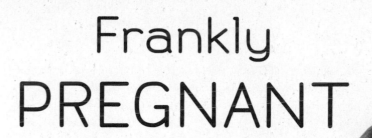

A Candid, Week-by-Week Guide to
the Unexpected Joys, Raging Hormones, and
Common Experiences of Pregnancy

Stacy Quarty
with Miriam Greene, M.D.

St. Martin's Griffin
New York

www.stmartins.com

Author photographs by Peter Hill, East Quogue, New York

Book design by Michelle McMillian

Library of Congress Cataloging-in-Publication Data

Quarty, Stacy.
    Frankly pregnant : a candid, week-by-week guide to the unexpected joys, raging hormones, and common experiences of pregnancy / by Stacy Quarty with Miriam Greene.
        p. cm.
    ISBN 0-312-34727-8
    EAN 978-0-312-34727-7
    1. Pregnancy. 2. Prenatal care. I. Greene, Miriam. II. Title.

RG525.Q37 2006
618.2—dc22   2005044454

First Edition: April 2006

10 9 8 7 6 5 4 3 2 1

For my mother,
who wasn't afraid to tell me
where babies really come from

A Note to the Reader

This book is intended to be used for informational purposes only and is not meant to replace the advice of your obstetrician or other medical professionals. Readers are advised to consult a trained medical professional before acting on any of the information in this book.

Contents

Contents

Acknowledgments

First, I want to thank all of my girlfriends and relatives who shared their most intimate, scary, humiliating, funny, and wonderful experiences of pregnancy and childbirth. I've created aliases for each so you won't be able to track down who insisted that her husband examine her hemorrhoids for fear it was the baby's first poking out. Thanks again to (real names): Kim, Lucia, Caroline, Debs, Burkley, Kelly, Mary, Susan, M.E., Nancy, Christina, Laura, Rosie, Donna, Bunky, Emily, Diane, and Erika.

Thank you to Jamey, my husband, who supported my nonpaying career as a writer trying to get published and never doubted (for the most part) that I would.

Kisses and love to my cherubs, Karmen and Devon, who have brought me more joy than I ever could've imagined and without whom this book couldn't have been possible.

I am eternally grateful to Dr. Miriam Greene, who agreed to jump on this haywire baby-birthing-bandwagon book and lend her medical expertise, humor, and support. When we first met, I asked her professional advice on "how to get pregnant," one of the most frequently asked questions on FranklyPregnant.com. She quipped, "Put the penis in the vagina!" I knew we were a great match!

I send a tremendous thank-you to everyone who visited my Web site, FranklyPregnant.com. Some shared stories or submitted questions and others sent glowing, inspiring letters of endorsement for my Web site and book project. These letters have been my greatest source of inspiration and have kept me plugging away at times when my enthusiasm and confidence were not at their highest.

The Herstory writing group helped me to shape my manuscript as my maternal shape expanded each month. Although some of the members had never, and would never, experience pregnancy, the support, feedback, and inspiration these ladies provided proved to be an indispensable tool in the birthing of this book. Thank you Erika, Linda, Marsha, Leslie, Peg, Lovey, Diane, Pat, Janessa, Tina, and Karen. For more information on this not-for-profit writing group, go to www.herstorywriters.org.

Thank you to Susan Schwartz, who pointed me in the right direction when I asked her, "How do I write a book? How do I get published?"

In the publishing world I also need to thank Lindsey Pollak, who's been there from the birth of FranklyPregnant.com. Also, thank you to Linda Konner, my agent, Sheila Curry Oakes, my editor, and Courtney Fisher, my publicist.

Last, I need to thank you, my fellow pregnant pal. Just like an ovum needs a sperm, without you, this book would never be possible.

Foreword

Pregnancy is a life-altering journey where only the fertile female can go, and if she chooses, she can take this trip multiple times. But no matter how many pregnancies a woman has, the path will never be exactly the same. On this path to becoming a mother she will encounter changes she never imagined possible in her body, in her shape, and with her emotions. Her belly will grow and swell. Her rings won't fit. Her shoes will be too tight. She will laugh at the silliest joke or cry during a sappy commercial.

As an obstetrician, I have the opportunity to travel alongside my pregnant patients. I offer guidance and advice along the road. Sometimes I simply hold a hand and bring comfort. At others I offer medical expertise in order for her to reach her destination safely.

Frankly Pregnant invites readers to follow along Stacy Quarty's pregnancy path and share her experience as well as those of some other women who have made this journey. The book is written in a lighthearted and humorous style, which can bring comfort and information to mothers-to-be. *Frankly Pregnant* also emphasizes the physiological and psychological importance of keeping a healthy outlook throughout pregnancy. It's important to laugh at yourself every now and then.

At the end of her fantastic journey lies the realm of mother-hood. It is where the hopes and dreams she has incubated for nine months become the life that will embody these hopes and dreams.

Miriam Greene, M.D.

Introduction

My friend Caroline recently reminded me that I've been sharing the real facts of pregnancy and childbirth since the age of seven.

At that time I found a compelling photo on the cover of a *Life* magazine in my parents' bookshelf. It was a picture of a bluish, slimy baby just coming out of the birth canal. Inside the magazine was a pictorial essay detailing conception, pregnancy, and childbirth. I was shocked to see a woman's vagina stretched to the limits with a misshapen baby's head peeking out.

The images brought many questions to mind. First and foremost, if a man's sperm fertilizes a woman's egg and the baby grows in the mother's belly and then comes out of the vagina, how does the sperm get in there? I had to ask my mother.

Initially she claimed I was too young to ask these questions. My pleading finally wore her down and we had the "talk." I learned that the man puts his penis inside the woman's vagina to insert the sperm.

"EEEEEEEEEEWWWWWWWWWWWWWWWWWWWWWWW WWWW!!!!!"

I could not wait to share the fascinating, scary, miraculous, and disgusting news with my friends. I called a neighborhood meeting. With the magazine as a visual aid, I spilled all the dirty details. A dozen ponytailed heads with wide marble eyes were fixed on the pages of the magazine as I relayed the story. I closed with the pizzalike afterbirth picture.

There were a few moments of silence before Caroline exclaimed, "That's not true! Babies come out of your butt, not your vagina." There was no convincing her otherwise, even with photographic proof. Her mother told her that babies came out of your rear end, very much like a big poo.

A week later, I was at Caroline's house playing dolls. Her mother stormed into the room and glared at me. "Stacy, do you know how to make babies?" she bellowed. Shocked and confused, I looked into the eyes of the plastic Baby Alive in my arms. Was she talking about dolls? Again, she taunted, "Do you know how to make babies?"

"Uh, no."

"Then don't go around telling my daughter lies about how babies are born!"

Caroline recently sent me a thank-you note for informing her about where babies really come from. She's due in about two months and claims she would have been really embarrassed at the hospital if she had listened to her mother's advice.

After delivering two of them myself, I'm now fairly confident that I know "how to make babies." I look forward to sharing the fascinating, scary, and disgusting news with you!

The Ovulation Game

When contemplating pregnancy and parenthood, we usually have an ideal image of how and when it should happen. My optimum plan for this, my second child, was to get pregnant at the end of the summer so the baby would be born in the spring. That way, I could take off the whole summer and enjoy the new baby.

With my first pregnancy I was never thinking that far ahead. It felt like we were trying for so long that just getting pregnant was all I could focus on . . . until it happened.

As you (probably) already know, when it comes to conception, things hardly ever work out as planned. My friend Bridget told me that not one of her four pregnancies fit into her "plan."

My husband, Jamey, and I had some major setbacks that delayed our pregnancy schedule by months. He had to take a few business trips during ovulation; I contracted a tick-borne disease; I had to have a minor surgery.

We finally had some normal months schedulewise but still no pregnancy.

Some couples get pregnant without ever really "trying," while others take years to conceive. If you fall into the latter category, you know as well as I that "trying" can become tedious and even stressful at times. Copulation on command is quite a feat. Everyone says the best thing to do is relax and forget about it. Ha! I don't know about you, but I spent many nights with my pelvis elevated by pillows, blood rushing to my head, and a constant chant droning in my head, "Go, sperm, go!" Far from relaxing, I assure you!

In early October we decided to go to the West Coast to visit some friends and attend a wedding. We were going to take a week's vacation and leave Karmen with my parents . . . and I would be ovulating! The trip was great. We were relaxed and had plenty of romantic time together (hotel sex), and I got to cuddle our friends' newborn baby. I'm not sure if there is any truth to the old wives' tale that handling a newborn can help get you pregnant, but it worked for me!

When we got back from our trip I could not wait to take a pregnancy test. I was sure that I was pregnant. I felt a presence, a life inside of me that was beginning to grow. Where this knowing feeling came from, I'm not sure. One girlfriend of mine said that she knew she was pregnant from the immediate physical feeling of tightness in her uterus. Another girlfriend told me that her knowing of conception was more spiritual. I would say that my "feeling" lay somewhere in between the physical and the spiritual.

I checked my calendar and did an "early response" test. It was negative. This could not be. How could my feeling be so wrong? Why wasn't I pregnant? Maybe I wasn't ever going to get pregnant. I used the second test in the kit. Still negative. Not pregnant.

The next night I went to dinner with a girlfriend and consumed more fluids than food. I was surprised to find myself quite drunk by the time dessert arrived. Almost every one of my girlfriends who has borne a child has had at least one (if not several) episode of alcohol consumption during early pregnancy—mostly because she had no idea she was pregnant. It also seems that lots of people get pregnant while on vacation, which lends itself to the more than occasional cocktail.

If you are recently pregnant and mentally flogging yourself for an incidental cocktail or two, try to let it go. After all, what's done is done. I'm sure you already know it's wise to abstain from the use of alcohol (and drugs) during and even prior to pregnancy to help produce the healthiest baby possible. (Remember, I don't claim to be an expert and this is by no means a clinical book. If you are concerned about your drinking habits before or after conception, see a doctor immediately.)

A week after my drunken dinner, I still did not get my period. That's strange, I thought. I checked my calendar and noticed that I had miscalculated my period due date. Whoops! I discovered that I was not alone in miscalculating. My friend Samantha had miscalculated her period due date by six weeks, if you can believe that! Her first indication of pregnancy was a nasty bout of morning sickness that she had mistaken for the flu. Surprise, surprise!

My period was definitely late this time, so I took the test again. Positive. What?! Positive! Am I ready for this?! Can I give up my body? Is our house big enough? Do we have to move? How will this affect my graphic design career? How will this affect my daughter? How will this affect my marriage? These and a zillion other questions consumed my brain. Of course I had considered all of these subjects on the road to this planned pregnancy, but now these issues were immediate and real.

After I calmed down, I was happy . . . and dying to tell someone. I couldn't wait for Jamey to get home from work. After all, he should be the first to know. Right?

I e-mailed him to ask what time he would be home. I planned to make a nice dinner and give him the news. He replied, "Sorry. Have a meeting directly after work. Won't be home 'til late."

Arrrrrrrggggggggghhhhhhhhhhhh! I needed to tell someone! I was bursting!

As it turned out, he did get home at a reasonable hour and I was able to share the news. I wrapped up the positive pregnancy test in a small, narrow box with silver paper and a red ribbon. Spying the gift on the kitchen table, two-year-old Karmen grabbed it and tried to unwrap it, assuming it was meant for her. I explained that it was a present for Daddy, a gift that only mommies could give to daddies but we could say it's from both of us. I'd let her give it to him when he got home.

The sound of the garage door alerted Karmen of Jamey's arrival. She grabbed the present, ran to the basement door, and began a dance of excitement and anticipation as she listened to him climb the stairs.

The moment he walked in the door, Karmen thrust the gift at him and squealed, "Open, now! Open, now!" Jamey opened the gift, with a quizzical look in his eye. Seeing the positive test, he was excited and delighted—a big change from his reaction to our first pregnancy, when he almost threw up.

You'd be surprised, but some men become quite queasy when contemplating the responsibilities of fatherhood. I guess that's the closest they will ever come to morning sickness! I wish I could say the same for me and many of my friends.

How *Sex and the City* Assisted in the Delivery of *Frankly Pregnant*

Although I don't consider myself a big television watcher, one of my favorites is HBO's *Sex and the City*. When I watch, I don't take phone calls, answer the door, or give more than one-word responses to questions asked of me.

One evening, after turning off the ringer on the phone and settling down with a large glass of ginger ale, I found that I had trouble paying attention to my show. Miranda's story line in particular reminded me of my own situation. I was newly pregnant and embarking on this book. Miranda was about to give birth on this very episode. It got me thinking, how could I deliver this book into the world without the proper assistance? I was certainly no medical expert and I needed someone to authenticate and contribute medical content.

"Okay, Miranda, go!" Dr. Greene said. After a few moments (remember this is a TV birth!), the baby was born. "He's perfect!" Dr. Greene exclaimed as she handed the nurse baby Brady.

She's perfect too, I thought. Dr. Greene, or someone like her, could help me deliver *Frankly Pregnant* into the world. So my quest to find that perfect OB/GYN began.

A few months later, a client of mine was telling me how much she enjoyed going to her OB/GYN. Strange, I thought. Most people dread it. "Dr. Greene has the most wonderful sense of humor and a very frank outlook," she went on. "I think you two would get along fabulously. Maybe she could help your book."

As luck would have it, she was the Dr. Greene from *Sex and the City*!

I contacted her, we clicked immediately, and she has been instrumental in giving medical advice throughout this book.

The book is taken from a journal I kept while pregnant with my second child and that I always intended to share with you, my pregnant pal. While I've already been through the experience, I left the journal in present tense so you can see the parallels of your pregnancy with mine. Keep in mind that we may have lots of similar experiences or only a few. It just goes to show you that no two pregnancies (even in the same woman) are alike. At the very least you may find yourself saying, "Thank God I'm not alone." Or, when you hear about some of my experiences or those of my friends, "Thank God that's not happening to me!"

Enjoy the journey!

Part One

. . . .

THE WEEKLY JOURNAL

1

Welcome to the Club

Pregnant? Me too! Congratulations!

Are you still in shock? I know I am.

I think I've been slightly stunned since getting a positive reading on the pregnancy test. I was in such a rush to get to work the day I took the test that I didn't wait for the result to develop and left the test in the bathroom. I was almost positive that I was not pregnant. I had already taken a pregnancy test a week prior, which was negative. While quickly cleaning up the bathroom before leaving the house, I almost swept the pee stick into the wastebasket. That's when I noticed there was more than one line. Positive? What?! I'm pregnant!

Can you believe it? We're pregnant! There is actually a microscopic life growing inside of us, and we are soon going to become someone's mother! Egads!

Before we get to the drama and implications of parenthood, we have a whole ten months of pregnancy to contend with. (Yes, *ten* months. 40 weeks: 9 months + 3 weeks = 10 months, at least in my book!)

So, what do we do now?

When I discovered my first pregnancy three years ago, I remember that my mind became frantically cluttered with questions: What was this pregnancy going to do to my life? What was it going to be like to "be" pregnant? Were people going to look at me differently? Were my feet going to grow? Was I going to get stretch marks? How much does childbirth really hurt?

Being a planner, I made a detailed list of everything I thought I needed to know and set out to find the answers.

During that first pregnancy I bought and faithfully read all of the standard pregnancy books: *What to Expect When You're Expecting, Your Pregnancy, The Girlfriends' Guide to Pregnancy, The Everything Pregnancy Book, Pregnancy and Childbirth,* the gory yet interesting *A Child Is Born,* and so on. These books were very helpful, but I felt I needed more. I wanted to know everything about pregnancy—from the most intimate physical changes to the psychological roller coaster I'd heard it could be. I wanted to hear every single detail from someone experienced and not afraid to discuss the various states of the vagina during pregnancy.

I questioned my doctor, my sister, my mother, and all of my closest girlfriends about their pregnancy and childbirth experiences.

I enrolled in the standard classes: Lamaze, Childbirth & Infant Care 101, and a pregnancy relaxation course.

After I completed all of my research, I still felt that many pertinent details had been omitted—by the books, by the doctors, and even by my own sister!

These details, sometimes quite gross or embarrassing in nature, are important for every pregnant woman to know (at least in my opinion!). For example: No one ever told me that I might feel baby hiccups in my rectum, that my nipples were going to crack apart into dozens of small sections that resembled dried desert mud, or that I would automatically earn a "pregnancy card" that would be handy when cutting in front of a hundred people waiting to use a public toilet.

You too probably have a gazillion questions about what to expect from your pregnancy. Some of your questions may be answered by your doctor or by reference books. Others may be answered by relatives or experienced maternal girlfriends.

With this book, a journal of my second pregnancy, I hope to help fill the gaps in between, and I promise not to withhold all of those "gory details." I will tell you when I wet my pants in public, what my body (and relationship) went through, and the story of my third nipple. Yup, third nipple.

My purpose is to give you, my dear reader and fellow pregnant pal, as much info as possible about pregnancy and childbirth—dirty details and all—while omitting most of the standard textbook stuff.

Be warned: I am sometimes brutally blunt and explicit (not for the dainty mannered gal). If you share my mentality and really enjoy a good "Ewwwww! Really?" among girlfriends, then read on!

If you have never given birth, the pain of labor and delivery may be your biggest fear. Before my first child was born I had envisioned the pain to be so encompassing that I feared I would lose my mind. I had been told many horror stories of women punching doctors, biting husbands, and spit-fit cursing the nurses.

I am happy to report that my brain (and saliva) remained intact during my delivery, and I knew I would gladly go through it all again to have another child.

Some people say that a mother forgets the pain of childbirth once it is over. I'm not so sure this is true. If you want to know what it's really like in the moment, I'm going to give you the real story.

I will document the birth of my child, blow by blow. I will have a laptop in the delivery room as well as a tape recorder to chronicle my various states of pain and sanity. I promise not to edit!

During my first pregnancy I remember thinking, Wouldn't it be fun to have a girlfriend who was pregnant and due about the same time, so we could share the experience and compare notes? I could ask her questions such as, "Are your boobs as sore as mine?" and "Do you have an equal ratio of skin tags to pills on your sweater?" I wrote this book so you can have what I didn't— a week-by-week chronicle of the hormonal highs and lows and everything in between.

I hope that by sharing my experience with you I may give you a more personal insight into the real experience of pregnancy and giving birth.

Keep in mind that not all women have the same experience and not all pregnancies are alike (even within the same person). If you are not having the same symptoms as I am, or even if you are experiencing something entirely different, it does not mean that you are abnormal. The range of what pregnancy symptoms you experience and when is vast. My friend Carol had morning sickness for the first three months; Abby never had morning sickness; Caroline was ill for the entire pregnancy. Guess what? All of these cases are considered "normal" for pregnancy.

If you're ever concerned about unusual symptoms, just ask your doctor or midwife. Some questions that came up for me and some of the women who logged onto the Web site include:

How is it possible there's enough fluid surrounding the baby when my vagina is leaking like a sieve?

So, is it normal to be limber enough to join Cirque du Soleil?

What is this sticking out of my butt?

Chances are, your doctor has heard that very same question many times before and your weird symptom is within the "realm of normality." And remember, the "realm" is very, very big!

One more thing. If you are one of those women who have an absolutely wonderful pregnancy every step of the way without a single discomfort or unpleasantry, well, cheers to you! Consider yourself doubly blessed.

I tend to be a bit of a complainer. I enjoy sharing my present states of discomfort and oddities with close friends. The daily reality of being pregnant, in my opinion, is not always a glowing miracle. Although it may be ugly at times, it can also be hilarious!

By the time you are finished reading this book, I hope that you may find the humor in a hemorrhoid and laugh when you break water on your mother-in-law's brand-new Persian rug.

Throughout this book you will notice that I quite often discuss (and complain about) the multitude of pregnancy symptoms I am experiencing. Here's a list of symptoms I had. This is by no means a comprehensive or definitive list. You may get a few of these symptoms. You may get none of these. You may get all of them and more. Who knows? Every pregnancy is so different, but it is fun to compare (and commiserate over) our stories.

SYMPTOMS OF MY PREGNANCY—THE UNEDITED LIST

Abdominal muscle separation. A separation can occur in the muscles of the abdomen from the pressure of the expanding uterus. This may be sore and accompany an umbilical hernia, or you may not notice it until after pregnancy.

Baby mambo. It can feel like your baby is doing the mambo from all the jabbing, kicking, poking, and squirming going on.

Backache. In early pregnancy it can seem like PMS back pain. By the last trimester it may be feeling more along the lines of a fractured spine.

Bleeding gums. Mucous membranes in the body become swollen and sensitive, including the gums. Even when brushing very carefully, your gums may bleed.

Bloating. Excess gasses and fluid retention can lead to frequent feelings of being bloated or overstuffed.

SYMPTOMS OF MY PREGNANCY—THE UNEDITED LIST

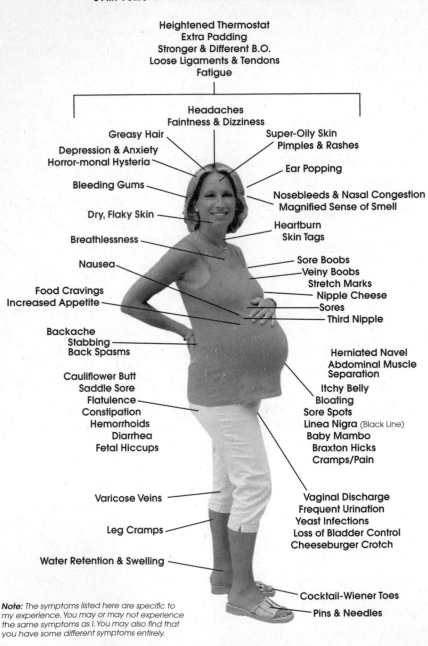

Heightened Thermostat
Extra Padding
Stronger & Different B.O.
Loose Ligaments & Tendons
Fatigue

Headaches
Faintness & Dizziness

Greasy Hair
Depression & Anxiety
Horror-monal Hysteria

Super-Oily Skin
Pimples & Rashes

Ear Popping

Bleeding Gums

Nosebleeds & Nasal Congestion
Magnified Sense of Smell

Dry, Flaky Skin

Heartburn
Skin Tags

Breathlessness

Nausea

Sore Boobs
Veiny Boobs
Stretch Marks
Nipple Cheese
Sores
Third Nipple

Food Cravings
Increased Appetite

Backache
Stabbing
Back Spasms

Herniated Navel
Abdominal Muscle
Separation

Cauliflower Butt
Saddle Sore
Flatulence
Constipation
Hemorrhoids
Diarrhea
Fetal Hiccups

Itchy Belly
Bloating
Sore Spots
Linea Nigra (Black Line)
Baby Mambo
Braxton Hicks
Cramps/Pain

Varicose Veins

Vaginal Discharge
Frequent Urination
Yeast Infections
Loss of Bladder Control
Cheeseburger Crotch

Leg Cramps

Water Retention & Swelling

Cocktail-Wiener Toes
Pins & Needles

Note: *The symptoms listed here are specific to my experience. You may or may not experience the same symptoms as I. You may also find that you have some different symptoms entirely.*

Braxton Hicks. These contractions can feel like menstrual cramps, intensified and then spread over the whole uterus. It reminded me of the crampy/nauseous/sweaty feeling one gets right before a bad bout of diarrhea. These contractions are quite common and normal for women in their third, and sometimes even second, trimester.

Breathlessness. Not only is the baby squeezing the space for your lungs, but the placenta is drawing oxygen out of your blood. If you overexert yourself, you'll be the first one shorted on the oxygen supply, not the baby.

Dr. Miriam Greene says: Your hormones also change the shape and capacity of your lungs during pregnancy.

Cauliflower butt. This is a result of multiple hemorrhoid eruptions. If you've got three or more hemorrhoids and they become irritated and inflamed, your anus may end up looking like a piece of purple cauliflower.

Cheeseburger crotch. The vaginal area becomes engorged with blood and fluids. My friend Grace and I fondly coined the term "cheeseburger crotch," because that's what it looked like she had stashed in her panties during pregnancy!

Cocktail-wiener toes. Retention of fluids in the lower extremities can leave you with toes that resemble overcooked cocktail wieners.

Constipation. Constipation during pregnancy is due to the fact that a mother's body draws and retains more fluids for the growing baby, placenta, and amniotic fluid, therefore making the stool dry. A dry stool has a much more difficult time moving through the pipes than a lubricated one.

Cramps/pain. Uterine cramps and pains can happen for a number of reasons, such as a muscle spasm; stretching tendons or ligaments; the baby kicking your cervix, bowels, or spine; or **Braxton Hicks** contractions.

Depression and anxiety. These, among many other wacky mood swings, can strike at any time.

Diarrhea. Speed of digestion and production of digestive enzymes can vary drastically during pregnancy, making diarrhea a common occurrence. Unfortunately, frequent diarrhea can bring about masses of hemorrhoids too.

Dry, flaky skin. In contrast to those super-oily spots, the dry spots of skin can become so flaky that they produce a small snowstorm of skin when scratched.

Ear popping. Swelling and fluid retention in the ear canal can create an ear-popping or clogged ear sensation. This is especially bothersome while trying to have a telephone conversation.

Extra padding. An entire-body covering of extra fat and fluid. Even if you've never had it before, you could get hand fat, ankle fat, neck fat, and back fat.

Faintness and dizziness. Sudden feelings of light-headedness and dizziness. I often saw sparkly stars before my eyes when I stood up too fast.

Fatigue. The feeling of being very run-down and tired.

Fetal hiccups. It might first feel like gas, but once you notice a rhythm you'll know your baby has the hiccups. The fetus and even newborns frequently get these muscle contractions in the esophagus.

Dr. Miriam Greene says: Fetal hiccups, although they can be annoying, are a wonderful sign. They mean your baby's neurological system is mature.

Flatulence. A mother's body slows down food in the intestine so that she may suck up every last nutrient. All the while, the contents are fermenting and creating huge pockets of gas. When the baby kicks or squirms, this gas can uncontrollably expel.

Food cravings. These must-have-or-I-might-hurt-someone-type foods can be the same for the entire pregnancy or may change from month to month or even week to week.

Frequent urination. During pregnancy, a mother's body processes many more fluids to feed the baby and expel wastes from the fetus. It's no wonder you've got to pee ten times a night.

Greasy hair. It seems the oil glands everywhere in the body work overtime during pregnancy, and it really shows in the scalp. Stock up on the shampoo!

Headaches. They can vary from a slight pressure in the skull to a jackhammer in the brain.

Heartburn. With limited stomach space, overactive stomach acids, and a lax reflux muscle, it's no wonder heartburn plagues pregnant women. During my last trimester, I felt the contents of my stomach rising up in the back of my throat whenever I lay down to sleep.

Heightened thermostat. A general feeling of being too hot, especially while sleeping.

Hemorrhoids. Growing pressure in the pelvic region compresses veins, arteries, and blood vessels. A hemorrhoid is a varicose vein that pokes out through the muscle wall near the anus. It can become very uncomfortable, even painful.

Herniated navel. A small hole in the muscle wall in or around the navel can cause bits of innards to squish out, and boy, is it painful!

Horror-monal hysteria. A general feeling of heightened emotions and a very short fuse to anger and rage. (Be careful while driving—road rage can run rampant.)

Increased appetite. I found that eating for two was not only my duty but also a pleasure. No one questions a pregnant woman ordering two cheeseburgers, two shakes, and two fries just for herself.

Itchy belly. Sensitive skin, expanding dermis, and a body that reacts more extremely to allergens makes belly itching most prevalent in the third trimester.

Leg cramps. One of the major causes of leg cramps during pregnancy is dehydration. Maybe that's why they happen so often at night when you're not able to drink a pint of water per hour.

***Linea nigra* (black line).** Starts just under the navel and ends at the top of the pubic bone. The line seems to be a pretty good indicator of how ripe your melon may be. The more prominent and dark it is, the closer you are to giving birth.

Loose ligaments and tendons. Not only do they loosen and stretch to accommodate a growing middle, but they also get rubbery in other parts of the body. You may have trouble holding onto small objects or even navigating your way to the bathroom with your looser-feeling limbs.

Loss of bladder control. Pressure from an expanding uterus puts the squeeze on your bladder. Since you are expelling liquids at an accelerated rate, the bladder fills up much more quickly. It can get harder and harder to hold your urine as the months progress.

Magnified sense of smell. You'd think with the nasal congestion, just the opposite would be true, but it's not so. It seems like the volume on the olfactory sensor is turned way up during pregnancy.

Nausea. Usually lasts for only the first trimester or so but can be constant (day and night) for weeks at a time.

Nipple cheese. This cheesy substance is a buildup of sebaceous fluid and/or early colostrum that collects on the nipples.

Nosebleeds and nasal congestion. Mucous membranes become very swollen and sensitive during pregnancy. You may feel like you have a continual stuffy nose. Do be careful—if you blow frequently or too hard, you may end up with nosebleeds too.

Pimples and rashes. Since your body is prone to more allergies, your thermostat is heightened, and your sweat and oil glands are working overtime, it's no wonder you can be more prone to pimples and rashes just about anywhere on your body during pregnancy.

Pins and needles. When there's a temporary blockage of blood to an area of the body, you'll have that pins-and-needles feeling. During pregnancy, excess weight and fluids and a shifting baby can cause pins and needles to happen to various parts of the body on a daily basis.

Saddle sore. Once the baby drops and the head is engaged in the pelvis, you'll notice a tremendous amount of pressure on the bowels, bladder, and pelvic bones. It can feel like you've been horseback riding for two weeks straight.

Skin sores. Most women's skin becomes extra sensitive during pregnancy, and sores can crop up anywhere there is an irritation. I got a smattering of sores just under my breasts from the friction of my bra.

Skin tags. Similar in appearance to pills on a sweater but they're actually small bits of skin attached to your underarms, groin, neck, and/or eyelids.

Sore boobs. It's no wonder they're sore with all of the expansion going on during pregnancy. By my second trimester it felt like my boobs were made of lead, and it was more than uncomfortable to go braless.

Sore spots. The baby can put pressure on, kick, or jab an area of the uterus, making it sore. It can feel very much like an internal belly bruise.

Stabbing back spasms. Muscles in and around the back can suddenly spasm and cause shooting pain throughout the body. My spasms sometimes left me looking like I'd been struck by invisible lightning.

Stretch marks. The skin stretches to the limit and the connective fibers within can break—creating a scar or stretch mark. Chalk it up to one of the battle scars of motherhood, I always say!

Stronger and different BO. Body odors can become much more pungent and entirely different smelling.

Super-oily skin. It seems the oil glands everywhere in the body work overtime during pregnancy. I got more grease off my forehead in a day than from two slices of fresh-from-the-oven pizza.

Third nipple. Most women never know they have excess nipple tissue until they become pregnant. The hormones released during pregnancy can make it swell up like a tick. Apparently, it is fairly common for people to have excess nipple tissue within a vertical line of the breast from the clavicle to the hip.

Vaginal discharge. This discharge, called leukorrhea, gets heavier as the pregnancy progresses. Eventually, you may have to use a sanitary napkin, a panty liner, or tissues to absorb the increasingly abundant discharge.

Varicose veins. An expanding body requires more blood supply, increasing the size of veins and arteries. Blue, purple, or greenish varicose veins and spider veins may crop up on your legs, belly, and breasts.

Veiny boobs. Expanding breasts require more blood supply, increasing the size of veins and arteries. Blue, purple, or greenish veins can give your breasts a road-mappish appearance.

Water retention and swelling. During pregnancy, your body can retain excess water. Changes in your blood chemistry cause some fluids to shift into your tissue. Usually the lower extremities, such as the legs and ankles, swell the most.

Yeast infections. Excess heat, perspiration, and discharge in the vaginal area create a breeding ground for yeast infections, which can happen frequently during pregnancy.

2

Week Four, Bursting with News

> **Symptoms:** bloating, moodiness, vaginal discharge

Before we get started, I would like to clarify my weekly pregnancy calendar. As you can see, I have started this chapter with week four, when in reality I have just missed my period and discovered that I am pregnant. Therefore, I should be two weeks pregnant. Right? ·

The reason I have started with week four instead of week two is that when doctors calculate your due date, they start counting from the first day of your last period. Of course there is no way you could be pregnant then because, chances are, you wouldn't be ovulating for another twelve to fourteen days.

I always thought that week one of pregnancy started at conception, but this is not the case. So if the doctors want to tack on another two weeks, let them. Besides, it made me feel a little better knowing that I was farther along than I originally thought—less time to wait out the forty weeks! If you want to keep up with doctorspeak, as far as what to expect at the weekly milestones, it's best to stick with the forty-week schedule.

I'm feeling a little bloating in the gut area, with slight cramps. It almost feels like gas or the beginning of my period. My friend Grace felt a similar bloating, and every day for a month she thought for sure she was about to get her period before she realized she was experiencing a symptom of pregnancy, not PMS.

I've been slightly moody. I noticed my emotions were a little out of whack when I lost track of how many times I told Jamey to "Shut up!" today.

I've also noticed a small amount of discharge in my underwear. It's similar to ovulation discharge, if you're familiar with that. At this point, it is generally clear and slimy, but not so much to be uncomfortable yet. I remember this discharge from last time. It's called leukorrhea and it gets heavier as the pregnancy progresses.

There are a few things you can do to alleviate the discomfort, wetness, stains, and yeast infections caused by the discharge: Wear dark-colored or patterned underwear so stains won't show; avoid tight, crotch-suffocating clothing (unless, of course, you want to lay out the welcome mat for yeast infections); wear only cotton underwear; and change panties frequently as they become moist.

Eventually, you may have to use a sanitary napkin, a panty liner, or tissues to absorb the increasingly abundant discharge. (Don't worry, by that stage of the game, abundant discharge will seem like a minor blip compared to all of the other symptoms you will be experiencing!)

During my first pregnancy, I found that panty liners tended to trap in moisture and give me yeast infections. I resorted to using toilet paper. Every time I went to the john (which was all the time), I would insert a fresh, neatly folded rectangle in my underwear. By my seventh month, I was using about ten rectangles a day.

After inserting rectangle number four one Friday afternoon, I took a break from work and went to the bank. A long line of people with paychecks snaked out the door. When it was finally my turn to approach the desk and deposit my check, I felt dozens of impatient eyes burning holes in my back. Suddenly, the rectangle of TP shimmied down my leg and out of my pants. A man in a gray, pinstriped suit stepped out of line and, in one chivalrous movement, picked up the rectangle and handed it to me. I accepted it graciously and quickly folded over the stained tissue.

I stifled my hysteria, exited the bank, and bumped into a girlfriend in the parking lot. I could hardly contain myself enough to relay the story of what had really dropped onto the ground!

I am pregnant once again and quite pleased with myself! I cannot wait to share the news with our family and friends. I hate waiting and I don't want people to assume that I am getting fat when in fact I am pregnant. Not only do I have to conceal a growing belly, but I also have to disguise symptoms of morning sickness, fatigue, and moodiness. Do we really need to wait the entire recommended three months to tell people? After three months you begin your second trimester, which is, statistically, a safer time. Statistically, most miscarriages happen within the first trimester.

If I do tell people early and have a miscarriage, I will have the unenviable task of following a joyous announcement with bad news. This is the last thing I want, so I will try to wait. With this second pregnancy I am feeling more sure of myself and of the baby. With the first, most of my troubling thoughts came from fear of the unknown. Ouch! Is this premature labor? Is the baby going to be okay? This time around I am recognizing each new symptom with an, Oh yeah. I remember that.

> **Dr. Miriam Greene says:** Don't be fooled. Whether you've had one or ten pregnancies, each experience can be so different symptomwise.

Jamey and I have decided (for now) that we're going to tell only the immediate family and wait until the second trimester to tell the world. We will see if I can keep my big yapper shut!

When I called my parents to tell them the news, before we could finish the preliminary pleasantries of "How are you . . . ," my mother excitedly guessed that I was pregnant. The same thing happened when I called my sister, although I was desperately trying to be casual. Maybe some kind of genetic intuition clued them in.

It was quite a different story with my in-laws. I kept waiting for them to guess the news: when I commented that my pants no longer fit, when I munched on saltines all day long, when I requested ginger ale instead of wine with dinner, and when I burped loudly enough to put an adolescent boy to shame they remained clueless. When it came time for the traditional family toast, I raised my sparkling glass of ginger ale and toasted to "the second little bugger" (they always referred to my daughter as "the little bugger"). They finally got it and were thrilled to death.

I feel like I have a million things to do to prepare for this pregnancy. I've made the doctor's appointment (should be seven weeks along by then), told the family, and started writing this book. When and how are we going to tell two-year-old Karmen that she's going to be a big sister? I hope she will be as excited as we are about this pending sibling. Maybe I will wait until I start to show, so we will have something physical to talk about and I will be more confident that this pregnancy is a keeper.

It seems like the arrival of the baby is forever away, but I know from experience that the time goes by so fast. By my calculations, the baby is due July 7. In the heat of the summer! Aren't I going to be stunning in my bikini? Public beaches will probably not be a good idea and I will most likely stay at home in the privacy of my own backyard. Lakes, pools, and water parks could also prove to be embarrassing.

During my last pregnancy I ate *way* too much and gained well over forty-five pounds. (That's a lot for a petite frame like mine.) I remember one sweltering summer weekend when a friend was visiting. She was going through chemotherapy and had lost all of her hair. She said, "Just look at us! I'm bald. You're fat. We are *not* going to the beach!"

This time I am going to try to eat more sensibly. We shall see if the raging hormones weaken my willpower again.

Dr. Miriam Greene says: For most of my patients I recommend a weight gain of twenty-five to thirty-five pounds during the pregnancy.

Most of my regular pants are already too tight. I've just purchased a pair of beautiful brown suede pants and have hardly worn them. I feel as if I've got to get as much use as possible out of my current wardrobe before it is too late.

Some pregnant women, myself included, become a bit panicky about losing their figures and bodily freedoms. The thought of giving up your body for the purpose of another life, for nine—excuse me, ten—months can be quite a scare. Not only do you lose your body for that period of time, but who knows what kind of shape you are going to have when it's all over. Plus, you become physically restricted in so many ways. Pregnant women shouldn't eat sushi and most soft cheeses, drink alcohol, go skiing, or even ride a roller coaster. Other pregnant women do not give a hoot about their changing physical appearances, the daily discomforts, or the freedoms surrendered.

My friend Sharon told me, "Stop whining about your damn suede pants! You should be focusing on the thrill of being pregnant and the creation of new life." During her pregnancy, she purposely gained extra weight in her first trimester so she would show earlier and be able to wear maternity clothes.

Sharon did surprise me, though, when she became unusually distraught over one purple stretch mark! "Oh, well," I told her. "Chalk it up to the battle scars of motherhood."

3

Week Five, A Little Bit Pregnant

Symptoms: belly bloating, tender breasts, vaginal discharge

I'm most definitely getting more bloating in the waist area. It looks and feels as if my intestines are so full of gas they are about to burst. It's time to go through the closet, try on clothes, and put away some of my "thin" pants. So sad.

My breasts are starting to get quite tender. They are feeling a bit more sore than your average PMS boobs. This, too, I know will get worse before it gets better. Well, at least my deflated water balloons will be perking up again. Soon I will be able to say bye-bye to my extra-padded (extra-pathetic) push-up bras! FYI, before my first pregnancy I had perfectly perky 34C boobs. After, they were sagging sacks of 34A.

I breast-fed Karmen for six months, but I don't think that has anything to do with the sorry state of my boobs. In my opinion, it's all heredity. Breasts get stretched out during pregnancy and get no bigger from breast-feeding. Take a look at your mother's breasts (if you have access) to get an idea of how yours may turn out.

Dr. Miriam Greene says: Your breasts are actually at their largest during pregnancy.

I'm also experiencing more vaginal discharge than normal, so I think it's time to put away the good white underwear before it gets ruined. I also have to keep an eye out for those escapee tissues at the bank!

I am physically feeling a bit more pregnant this week but still cannot quite believe that I am. Half of my brain is telling me that my sore breasts are PMS, so just dismiss it. The other half of my brain is saying, "This is a real symptom of pregnancy. Remember, there is a baby growing inside of you."

I guess it is easy to forget (momentarily) that you are pregnant, when you don't yet have the large, cumbersome belly as a constant reminder. I'm sure my upcoming smorgasbord of symptoms will soon be my friendly daily reminders of my maternal condition.

I am trying to make the appropriate adjustments to my physical activity and diet. It is so hard to give up all of the things that pregnant women are not supposed to have and not supposed to do. For instance, I enjoy a nice glass of wine with dinner, and a few more on weekends. I also love a hot sake with a sushi dinner. I went to a Japanese restaurant last night, and it was such torture to have only the cooked stuff and a cup of green tea.

During my last pregnancy, I found the only thing that finally curbed my feelings of loss over certain foods and alcohol was the good ol' morning sickness. It must be nature's way of encouraging consuming a more bland diet to be safer for the baby.

If you are fortunate enough to skip the morning sickness, I hope you do not have too many pregnancy no-nos to give up. You'll have to do it with willpower alone.

As far as exercise is concerned, I am still keeping up with my morning run, although I do not do the long run on weekends anymore. Experts say more than twenty minutes of an elevated heart rate may take away oxygen from the baby.

Dr. Miriam Greene says: During exercise, you should try not to exceed 140 bpm (heartbeats per minute).

Pregnancy isn't a good time to take on a new strenuous exercise routine. If you are already exercising, you can continue to do so, as long as you inform your doctor of your activities and let your body tell you when to quit.

I have noticed my tendons and ligaments are getting a bit more rubbery, especially while doing my stretching, so I must be careful not to overextend. I don't remember at what point it comes about, but there was a time during my last pregnancy when all of my tendons and ligaments felt extremely loose.

Once during that last pregnancy, while in the supermarket, I slipped—literally—on a banana peel and almost did a split across aisle two. I had never been that limber before! I felt like a Barbie doll that had the legs taken off and put back into the sockets backward—very awkward indeed! Fortunately, there were no injuries. Even my pride was saved because no one saw me, but I was a bit sore in the groin afterward.

I had forgotten just how many little changes happen during pregnancy. Can't wait to see what thrilling new symptom is next!

4

Week Six, A Tiny Flicker

Symptoms: belly bloating, expanding breasts, tender breasts, morning sickness, dry skin patches, greasy skin and hair, food cravings, blood in vaginal discharge

I'm now getting more bloating in the midsection. I cannot believe it. I am already developing the "Buddha belly." I have heard that during the second pregnancy, the belly pooches out sooner. Oh, no! I don't know how long I can keep this secret with a protruding gut!

My breasts are expanding at an equal rate to the belly and getting increasingly sore. Running without a sports bra is definitely out of the question! I made that mistake one morning and ended up having to run while holding my boobs. I did have to release them occasionally when a car passed by.

Another discomforting symptom I am starting to experience is morning sickness. If you have this too, you probably already know by now that morning sickness is not limited to the morning. It can last all freaking day! Mine is not too bad yet, but I have had episodes of faintness, nausea, mouth watering, and weakness—usually on an empty stomach. I have been trying to eat small meals more often. It helps a little.

During my last pregnancy, I remember feeling most nauseous

when contemplating food choices. At a business lunch one day, I was trying to decide what to order. Hmmmm. Fried fish—greasy, scaly, smelly, . . . nauseating; pasta with sautéed tomatoes and garlic—acidy, slimy, garlic breath hell . . . nauseating; cheeseburger—greasy, heavy, meat funky smelling . . . nauseating; chicken soup— bland, light, boring . . . perfect! I opened my mouth to reply and produced a jarring, juicy burp. It must have reeked of stomach acids, because the waiter took two steps backward with the

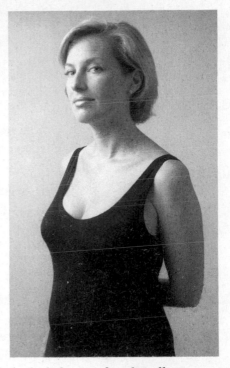

notepad over his face. I did feel a little better after dispelling some of my stomach gases. At the time, I thought it was worth the embarrassment to have a little relief from the gripping feeling of sickness.

It certainly is a lot easier to hide feelings of sickness than a really poor complexion. I am afraid that is what I may soon have, with all of the rapid changes happening to my skin. I've always had combination skin—dry with oily patches—but now each has become extreme. The skin by my mouth and chin is dry, flaky, and irritated, while my forehead and nose are an oil slick. Just yesterday, Jamey gave me a big, loving hug as we contemplated what this new baby will bring to our lives. When I pulled back, I noticed a large greasy stain on his white shirt. It's as if my forehead is producing olive oil! Not only is the skin on my face a nightmare, but my scalp is also breaking out. I am getting dozens of itchy zits on my head. The more I scratch at them, the greasier my hair gets.

This morning began with a good bout of lightheadedness and nausea. I wish I could have stayed in bed. My head nestled into my soft pillow and the blanket gently cocooned my tired and weakened body. I needed a few more minutes to drift off and . . .

"Mommy!" screeched Karmen. Abandoning my haven and staggering into her room, I was immediately assaulted by the smell of a poopie diaper. While changing Karmen, I had to take a break, put my head down, and wait for the faintness to pass.

Later, in the bathroom, I discovered that the discharge in my underwear was slightly brown when I wiped myself and inspected the toilet paper. I deduced that there was definitely blood. The sight of blood during pregnancy always sets off the alarm bells, although this happened during my last pregnancy too.

What could this blood mean? The beginning of a miscarriage? Is there something wrong with the baby? Is there something wrong with my uterus or the developing placenta?

From what I have read, all of these concerns are a possibility, but at what point do I call the doctor? How much blood does there have to be? What color does it have to be—brown or red?

Dr. Miriam Greene says: You should report *any* amount of bleeding during pregnancy to your OB/GYN, as it may indicate a problem.

I picked up the phone to call my obstetrician, then reconsidered. Should I wait until after lunch to call the doctor? Maybe by then the spotting will have stopped. Spotting happened during my last pregnancy too, and everything was fine. I put the phone down. But wait. What harm can it do to call the doctor? I'm sure I am not the only one to call with a seemingly unimportant question. Isn't it better to risk looking stupid than the health of the baby? I picked up the phone and dialed.

I have an appointment today at 2:45 P.M., two weeks earlier than I was originally scheduled to go in. The doctor is going to do an internal sonogram and has warned me that at five weeks it may be too early to detect a fetal heartbeat, so I should not be alarmed if we can't locate the heartbeat.

Honestly, I am looking forward to the appointment. I am glad to be going earlier than originally scheduled, and it would be exciting if I do get to see the baby's heartbeat!

The great news is: I saw it! I saw a tiny flickering of the baby's heart. At first, all that appeared on the sonogram was the dark circle of the yolk sac, but after a little maneuvering, the pea-sized baby made an appearance. There it is! There's the "little bugger." To actually see that there is a baby inside of me makes the pregnancy more real, more jarring, more permanent—more exciting.

Okay, the baby is still there. "What about the blood?" I asked. My doctor told me that, yes, blood can indicate a number of problems, but in this case we can see that the baby is alive and well, so I should not be too concerned. Although there may be no specific reason for it, bleeding in the first trimester can be completely normal.

After I was finished with the sonogram, the nurse gave me the RhoGAM shot. It prevents an Rh-negative mom like me from developing antibodies to the baby's blood if that turns out to be Rh-positive.

I am not fond of this shot. It's a little uncomfortable and the last time I almost passed out from it. This time was not quite as bad, but I still felt faint. Getting it in the butt instead of the arm probably helped.

Even though seeing the sonogram helped quell my fears and let me know I'm definitely pregnant, my recent cravings and strange eating habits are yet another confirmation that this baby is the real thing. Some women crave the same few items throughout their entire pregnancy. My friend Nicole had to have a mango bean burrito three times a week. She frequently sent her husband out in the middle of the night to acquire one of these treasures. I believe he deserved an honorary medal, especially since the restaurant that made them was more than thirty minutes away.

At this point, I think my cravings are changing on a daily basis. I have had hankerings for spicy Buffalo wings, coconut shrimp, yogurt, Jell-O, and everything bagels. I am gagging as I write this. To think of foods that I have had within the last forty-eight hours makes me want to puke. It's odd how much I can want a particular item, but sighting leftovers in the fridge is complete torture and makes me nauseous.

Dining out is becoming a little problematic as well. Restaurant menus seem so limiting: Why isn't my "craving of the day" listed here? Anyone who really knows me and shares a meal with me is going to be able to tell something is up. Not only are my orders fussy and unusual, but I am not drinking wine with dinner. The smell and taste of alcohol actually make me want to wretch. Oh, goody! I am over my desire for the "bad stuff."

Socializing also presents other problems. I cannot tolerate the smell of a single cigarette. I never have liked the smell of butts (ha ha), but the odor is extremely offensive now. The dial has been turned way up on my olfactory sensor. A smoky restaurant is completely out of the question. I find that even in establishments that have a separate smoking section, the smell gets to me.

I also am getting tired more quickly, especially after eating a meal. It feels similar to the tiredness one gets after taking a too-large dose of cold medication. Fighting it is pointless. People can tell from my glassy, droopy eyes, my lack of conversation, and my listless movements that I am ready for nighty-night.

Sleep seems so important these days. Each morning I stay in bed until the last possible minute, trying to savor every moment of glorious rest.

5

Week Seven, An Anxious Week

Symptoms: magnified sense of smell, morning sickness, poor complexion, more blood in vaginal discharge

My sense of smell has always been very keen, but this week it seems that my sniffer is even more sensitive than ever. Last night Jamey had a few beers while watching "the game," whatever it was. He came to bed and then assaulted me with his reeking, sour, yeasty alcohol breath. Every time he directed his noxious air in my direction, I was jolted awake by the feeling that I was going to throw up. The stench was so heavy and repugnant that even the ceiling fan didn't help remove it. I would have moved into the guest room if my body didn't feel so leaden.

My friend Hannah slept in another bedroom throughout her entire pregnancy. She said the smell of her husband's sleep/morning breath was so offensive she would vomit upon whiffing it. I wonder if her smell sensor was unusually heightened, or if his breath was really that deathly.

The morning after Jamey's beer breath assault, I was surprised by the fact that I did not feel as nauseous, noxious smells and all. I think the morning sickness may be waning. Oh, please, let it be so!

Although I still have bouts of nausea, I am able to eat more and have periods of actually feeling all right. I may be getting off too easily if this really is the beginning of the end of the nausea. We shall see.

I've noticed that my complexion is definitely getting worse. At first glance in the bathroom mirror, I found my dry patches so flaky that I could, with a few scratches, produce a small snowstorm of skin in the sink. I was tempted to take my toothbrush and slough off enough skin to create a tiny winter wonderland, but I thought better of it and went off to work.

After work that day I was shocked to see a tomato-sized stain of bright red blood in my underwear. I was terrified. Was the last bleeding episode just a precursor to the actual miscarriage?

Perspiration oozed from every pore as I called my OB/GYN. My doctor said it very well may be the beginning of a miscarriage. I was frightened, but I snapped to attention as he doled out the list of commandments for the weekend: no physical exercise or exertion, no sex, and no stress. (Ha! Easy for him to say.)

I was scheduled for another sonogram on Monday morning. There was nothing he could do for me until then. I would just have to wait and see. "Wait and see?!" I wanted to scream. The life of this baby was uncertain, and I would have to wait and see? How could he put it so casually?

As you can imagine, waiting the entire weekend was horrible torture. If it was a miscarriage, I wanted to know, and know right away. Was the tiny heart still beating or was it extinguished, soon to be discarded? I could already picture him as a toddler, giggling as I push him higher and higher on the swing under the crab apple tree.

If this was a miscarriage, I wanted to get through it and over it as soon as possible. If this wasn't to be, I needed to erase the visions of a million kisses on petal-soft chubby cheeks, tickles on wiggly pink toes, a small hand to hold, and a tiny orange-sized head to sniff.

Stop it, stop it, stop it. It can't be true that I'm going to lose this baby. The strange thing was that although my logical mind was telling me otherwise, something in my gut was telling me that the baby was okay.

"Look at the facts," logic said. "These are the symptoms of miscarriage."

"No. Don't listen. The baby is fine," an inner voice whispered. Who was that? My guardian angel?

Jamey was much more outwardly negative than I was. His concerned looks made me doubt my calm inner voice. Did he and logic have a point? Was I wrong? After all, it was two against one.

The bleeding continued, quite heavily, through Friday night and all day Saturday. It was as much blood as a normal period, and all very, very bright red. This could not be good. Chalk one up for logic.

I have never so carefully inspected the contents of my underwear. I kept checking the consistency for lumps, as that may indicate a miscarriage. Every time I looked I was slightly relieved to see there were no bits of tissue present. Chalk one up for the inner voice.

We had planned to have dinner at our friends' house that Saturday night. We were going to tell them the "good news" of our pregnancy in person. Everyone else in our small East Coast town already knew our secret. I told one friend, who is also newly pregnant. Jamey had to discuss our maternity insurance with someone in his office. It spread from there. Now everybody knows except some of our closest friends, whom we were going to tell this particular Saturday night.

We decided to tell our friends because we figured they would find out from someone else eventually. If it was a miscarriage, everyone else was going to know, so why not them too? With forced smiles on our faces, we relayed our "good" news. I played down our concerns over the massive amount of bleeding I was having and quietly sneaked off to the bathroom to change my pad.

On Sunday, the bleeding slowed down considerably. Whew! Finally, a sign of hope! Okay. The inner voice is back on top.

First thing Monday morning, I confirmed my appointment for the sonogram, dropped my daughter off at day care, and was on my way.

During the trip to the doctor's office, I envisioned how I might react if it was bad news. I decided that I would keep my composure, at least until I got back into the privacy of my own car.

My stomach was clenching painfully and my face was hot as I stepped into the doctor's office. While walking from the waiting area to the examining room, I felt as though I might pass out, so I steadied myself on the wall, plastered with pictures of newly delivered babies. Was *my* baby going to make "the wall"? I was telling logic to shut up as the doctor came in. I quickly uncreased my brow.

The doctor began with the preliminary chitchat. Let's get on with it, I thought. Are these pleasantries really necessary? Finally, the nurse blobbed some jelly onto the joystick and we were off. The doctor was quiet for quite a long time while looking at the monitor. From what I could tell, it looked like the yolk sac was still there and there was something inside it, but it wasn't moving. It looked twice as big as it did last time, but I did not see a heartbeat. There was no flickering.

After a few more "Hmmmmmms" the doctor told me everything looked fine and then directed the joystick at the baby so we could see the heartbeat. Whew! The baby was fine! The images of the toddler on the swing came into focus once again. The baby was alive! The doctor said at this point that my chances of miscarriage are only about 7 percent. That made me feel a whole lot better than the fifty-fifty chance I was given on Friday night.

It's true that bleeding in the first trimester can be perfectly normal, but it certainly is scary!

My friend Dana had a similar experience in her second month and actually saw small bits of lumpy tissue in the blood. She thought she surely had a miscarriage and was devastated. As it turned out, the baby was fine. Her doctor told her it might have been some kind of uterine hematoma her body was dispelling in the early stages of pregnancy.

Just remember, you never know until you can check with your doctor. Logic doesn't always have to win.

6

Week Eight, Baby Lima Bean

Symptoms: morning sickness, fatigue

I'm still having morning sickness. I must have been delusional to think that I was getting over it already. At this very moment I am munching on saltines and sipping ginger ale to quell the nausea. Burp!

I am also getting more tired with every passing day. Generally, by 3 P.M. I have had it. Napping a bit does help. Exhaustion becomes a real challenge to fight at the end of the day. Dragging limbs and heavy eyelids make preparing dinner an Olympic event.

Getting ready for a dinner party the other night seemed like the triathlon. I was chopping at a good rate for the food preparation. My whisking, sautéing, and basting were right-on. But by the third and final event, the presentation, I was so tired I could hardly lift a casserole dish. My pace slowed considerably and hindered the outcome. The turkey was too dry—I couldn't get it out of the oven soon enough—and the mashed potatoes (a new recipe) tasted like dirt. I should have known better than to try something different, especially with guests at the table.

I can't seem to get it together like I used to. Ah well, just chalk it up to one of the many "joys of it all."

Now that the scare of my bleeding episode is over, I am feeling much more calm and confident about this pregnancy. Being pregnant the second time around definitely is different from the first. It seems that my judgment about possible signs of trouble is much more clear. I no longer have anxiety over the unexpected—wondering if my seemingly strange symptoms are normal and, of course, stressing about how painful, scary, and possibly traumatic the actual birth will be.

Although I am now more relaxed, there is one thing that I do miss—the kind of

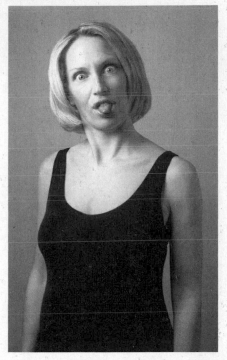

schoolgirl excitement, butterflies-in-the-stomach feeling one gets when experiencing something for the very first time.

With my first pregnancy, every new symptom wasn't an inconvenience or annoyance, but another reminder that I was actually going to have a baby. Yes, me. I was going to have a baby—a little person to hold and to love who was a part of me! Being pregnant for the second time is exciting, but you don't usually have the same butterfly feeling as you do with your first kiss, first crush, or first true love. If this is your first, revel in it. It is truly a once-in-a-lifetime experience!

I had my real "first visit" at the OB/GYN's today. The visit consisted of a battery of standard tests, another sonogram, and my first weigh-in. I wondered if I could gain the recommended twenty to thirty pounds from this weight forward, or if the recommended amount is based on the preconception weight. I didn't remember how it was done last time. I'll have to write that down so I don't forget to ask my doctor. (It's a good idea to have an index card or notepad of questions prepared for every OB/GYN appointment. You'd be surprised how easy it is for your mind to go blank while in the stirrups.) Unfortunately, I have to report that the weight gain starts being counted from your pre-conception weight. It's not fair!

Dr. Miriam Greene says: During an initial visit, I routinely do a full physical and gynecological exam plus a blood test, which screens for rubella, measles, toxoplasmosis, hepatitis B and C, CMV, HIV, diabetes, and anemia.

After hopping off the scale, I was actually looking forward to getting up on the table and into the stirrups for the internal sonogram. This time I had no worries or doubts about the condition of my baby.

Yep! There it was on the monitor, perfectly intact and flickering away. I again noticed some growth in the size of the baby. It is about the size of a lima bean. I got to bring home baby's very first picture from the sonogram. The lima bean is now pinned to our fridge, among dozens of other pictures of Karmen, family, and friends. Welcome to our life, little baby!

7

Week Nine, Getting a Grip

Symptoms: morning sickness, constipation, frequent urination, flatulence

My morning sickness comes and goes. Some days I feel energetic and well, while others I feel listless and pukey. I guess I am about fifty-fifty with the good and bad days. On one particularly bad day, I had to read some documents while being driven back from a late-day meeting. I was wearing a fairly snug turtleneck sweater and should have known better. A garment that warm and throat binding was far from helpful at battling nausea. By the time I returned to my own car, I was drenched in prevomitus perspiration. I took off my sweater and drove home in my bra. I drove a little too fast, as I wanted to get home before I threw up. I mentally dared a cop to pull me over. What chance would he have against a woman with pregnancy insanity?

Constipation made its first appearance a few days ago. I have been told that one of the best ways to conquer constipation is to answer the call of nature right away. Don't wait for even a minute, or you may miss your window of opportunity.

Constipation during pregnancy is due to the fact that a mother's body draws and retains more fluids for the growing baby, placenta, and amniotic fluid, therefore making the stool dry. You can try to conquer colon dehydration by drinking more liquids, but then you run the risk of increasing the already way-too-frequent urination problem. I have not mentioned frequent urination until now because, although frequent, it was not a big issue for me until recently. Last night I got up eight times for the toilet. How is a person supposed to get any sleep?

These bodily changes are a major reminder that my body no longer belongs to me exclusively. That "other someone" is getting most of the attention. It is clear that my comfort has taken a backseat to the baby. It's like I have handed over the master controls to someone else, and I don't really like the way that someone has been playing me.

My friend Grace, although well versed on the common symptoms of pregnancy, was quite surprised when she actually experienced them. "What have I got myself into now?" she moaned, white-knuckled, at the base of the "porcelain god." She never thought that pregnancy would be so debilitating.

While she was pregnant, I frequently shared with Grace all of the surprising and annoying symptoms of my first pregnancy. Did she really think all of my complaints were a severe case of hypochondria?

Now I am trying to gain some control over my symptoms and my body. Maintaining regular activities helps a little, like playing tennis. I have just started playing again for the first time in months. I had to cancel a few dates when I had the scare with the bleeding. My friend Bridget played tennis until the day she delivered. Although her tall, lean, and bulbous form was a funny sight to see in clingy tennis garb, I certainly did admire her skill and determination through those last few months. Barring physical setbacks or complications, I plan to try to play as long as she did. It may be tough to live up to such a shining example.

On my first day back playing tennis, I was pleasantly surprised by the fact that I felt good physically, and I did not give the baby a thought the entire time. Again, I am feeling much more energetic and nonnauseous. Tomorrow (a tennis lesson) will tell the tale—does exercise make me feel less pukey or not?

I'm pleased to report that exercise definitely helps me with the morning sickness and energy levels. Aha! I have gained some control! I hope exercise helps you too, if you are also struggling for your master controls.

Dr. Miriam Greene says: Remember to keep your doctor informed of your physical activities.

While exercise is curbing some symptoms, it's absolutely no help whatsoever in controlling my frighteningly loud flatulence. Apparently, the reason for frequent farting (and burping) during pregnancy is the slowness of digestion. A mother's body slows down food in the intestine so that she may suck up every last nutrient. All the while, the contents are fermenting and creating huge pockets of gas. It's got to come out one end or the other.

Just this morning as I rolled out of bed, I startled myself with a fart so boisterous it sounded like I had just ripped the sheets. My poor husband was horrified. Sorry, honey, you're going to have to get used to it! The morning gas is particularly hard to control.

I'm concerned that memories of my honking farts may linger in my husband's mind. Will this diminish his desire for me? Gas is not the only thing, I'm sure, that is stacking up negative points against my sex-appeal factor. There's also the blotchy and blemished skin; a widening rear end; extra deposits of cellulite; blue, veiny breasts with big, dark, shiny, bumpy, cracked, cheesy nipples; different and stronger body odor; and a darker and larger crotch. How can a body like this be sexy?

Hormones, physical changes, cultural values, and a husband's view on the pregnant body could all be contributing factors to a negative or a positive body image for oneself. If you happen to be feeling negative like I am this week, try to remember that pregnancy is not forever. One day you will have your body back to yourself, although it may be a little worse for the wear.

On the other end of the spectrum, some women feel more body positive and sexy as pregnancy progresses.

Marsha says she was never more confident in her physical appearance than when she was pregnant. She normally had low self-esteem when it came to the looks department. She hardly ever wore the negligees that her husband bought her for every anniversary. When she got pregnant, she wore the negligees so often that she stretched out or tore every piece she owned. My guess is that the torn negligee had more to do with her husband's enthusiasm than her expanding girth!

Nicole's husband, too, was quite content sexually when she was pregnant. The surge of hormones heightened her sex drive to such a level that he never complained of not "getting enough." Not only that, he says he enjoyed her larger, more voluptuous body for a change. (For more good news on "pregnancy sex," see Week 21.)

Bridget's husband, although an apparent sex maniac, rarely wanted intercourse during her pregnancy. He claimed his biggest fear was that his "oh-so-large penis" would hurt the baby.

I suppose this is a genuine concern men have. However, everything I have heard from doctors and read in books leads me to believe that this fear is purely nonsense. Sure, intercourse during risky times (bleeding episodes or placenta previa cases) is not recommended, but for the most part it is perfectly healthy. Intercourse at the very end of pregnancy may even stimulate the softening of the cervix and the beginning of labor—which is a good thing, believe me. Take it from one who was ten days overdue!

Although you may have the desire, most of my girlfriends agree that by the end of the forty weeks it's hard to convince your mate to have sex with you. He may not be as attracted to your physical form, he may fear hurting you or the baby, plus he will have to do most of the work. There really is not much more you can do than just lie there and graciously accept your . . . sexual pleasuring.

8

Week Ten, Starting to Show, Starting to Stink

Symptoms: acne, different and stronger body odors, pooching belly, diarrhea

Acne! I can't believe that I have acne again. I thought adolescence was the last I'd see of it. I'm seeing a new crop of zits sprout up every night—along my hairline and my jawline, in my scalp, and on my chest and back. I planned on wearing a scoop-neck dress to a party I will be attending this weekend, but I'll be nixing that outfit. I don't think I need to spotlight my skin eruptions.

I tried covering the pimples with makeup, but it only made matters worse. It reminded me of the time when I was in junior high at the roller rink and I tried to cover up a festering zit with a cover stick that was way too orange. I thought it looked okay in the dimly lit bathroom, but when I went to meet the cute boy who had asked me to skate, I knew something was awry when he couldn't stop staring at what I later found to be a large, orange mound on my chin.

Now I am puffy, greasy, and zitty. What else could there be? Oh, yes—now I am smelly too. While getting undressed last night, I wondered, What is that smell? The dog? Did she roll in something? As I picked up my clothes off the bed, I smelled it

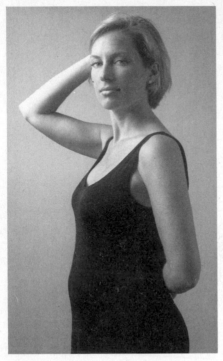

again. I whiffed my shirt. Ack! That smell is me!

My bodily odors are decidedly different from before pregnancy. I've been noticing a gradual change, but now I think I smell like a whole new (and not so fresh) me. My BO smells muskier than it used to, and not only do I smell different, but also I smell stronger. During my last pregnancy, I remember resorting to taking two showers a day. This may have to go into effect very soon, and I'm only newly pregnant. By the end of my ten months, will I be showering four or five times a day? Who has that kind of time?

I am happy to report that today I am feeling fine. I'm slowly getting over the morning sickness and am back to tennis a few times a week. Hooray! I wonder how long I'll be able to keep it up before my belly starts getting in the way.

The belly is definitely getting more noticeable. In the morning

Dr. Miriam Greene says: About 30 percent of pregnant women experience morning sickness of some kind. It can range from a mild sickness to extreme nausea where the patient is unable to ingest sufficient amounts of nourishment and must get medical attention. The good news is that most moms-to-be are better by fourteen weeks.

it's fairly small, but by 3 P.M. it is out in full force. Jeans that I was able to comfortably zip up at the start of the day are completely unzipped by evening, with no chance of closing more than two teeth together. The late-day belly is so much bigger than the early A.M. pooch.

We went to a party last night, and people who knew that I am prego said they noticed the pooch. Remember, at this point we have decided to tell only family and close friends. On the one hand, I was proud to finally be showing—"Hey, I'm going to be a mother. There's really a baby in there." On the other, I was a bit self-conscious, wondering what other people must be thinking—Maybe she's bloated with gas? and Oh, she's really losing her shape. Can I really wait five more weeks to tell everyone?

I was so relieved actually to be feeling nonnauseous that I overindulged at the party. Not drinking, mind you, but food. There was a glorious buffet set up with smoked salmon, roast beef, lobster, escargot, shrimp cocktail, four kinds of pasta, grilled vegetables, five kinds of salad, puffed pastries, sinful brownies, two kinds of cake, and three fruit pies—and none of it made me queasy!

After feeling sufficiently stuffed, I settled into my seat and began to notice a warm sensation coming over my face and neck. Shortly after, stomach cramps set in. Oh, no! I thought as I made a mad dash to the bathroom in this very tiny restaurant.

Fortunately, I made it on time but then suffered through a bout of stomach-wrenching diarrhea. The smell was so foul it was making me even more sick to my stomach. All the while, some woman was persistently knocking on the door. Oh, please just quit the room-jarring knocking and go away! I thought. I am dying in here!

When I finally emerged several minutes later, she was knocked right over with the smell! Oh, gosh! Is there some dark closet I can go hide in?

That was a lesson to be learned. It seems that every time I eat too much, I get diarrhea. I will have to be much more careful, especially in public places!

9

Week Eleven, Mistaken for Fat

Symptoms: headaches, pooching belly

I was so happy finally to be over the morning sickness, but that didn't last for long. The nausea has been replaced with constant headaches. My head feels like I have a sinus pressure–induced vise on my skull. When I sleep at night, I usually lie on my right side until that side of my head becomes so congested and headachy that I have to roll over. I feel like I'm doing the flip-flop all night long to even out my skull pressure.

I am very prone to migraines, which these terrible headaches can easily escalate into. As a matter of fact, it happened just yesterday. The constant throbbing in my skull transformed into a debilitating, knife-stabbing pain by the end of the day.

I normally take a prescription medication for the migraines, but now my options are very limited. Tylenol just doesn't cut it. I do remember from last time being able to take small doses of another prescription drug for my migraines. I have to get my hands on some of that—and soon. I have a call in to the doctor now with a query about my pain relief options.

Dr. Miriam Greene says: Some medications are perfectly safe, but consult your doctor before taking any drugs during pregnancy.

Like my migraines, you may find that some of your chronic problems may give you more trouble during pregnancy. My sister-in-law had injured her tailbone a year before she became pregnant. She always found it to be a bit sore, especially during her menstrual cycle. When she became pregnant with twins, she said she felt as if the injury was more painful than the first day she fell on her rear end.

I have officially been mistaken for fat now. Yes. This is one of the many humiliations we pregnant ladies must endure. I was at a wedding this past weekend, wearing a semiclingy dress that really showed the little pooch and my nonexistent waistline. After conversing with a friend whom I hadn't seen in several months, the subject of my pregnancy came up. (By the way, we are telling people now. I just can't keep the secret any longer!) She audibly sighed and exclaimed that she and her husband thought that I had put on a few!

I wonder why the waistline is the first to go. Maybe the expanding uterus pushes the other organs to the left and the right first, before squishing them up and out? The look of the nonwaist is so odd—just like that of an adolescent boy, but with a gut.

The protruding gut is starting to push out my already deformed belly button. Before my first pregnancy, I had a navel so deep that I could never see the bottom. At the end of the pregnancy, my belly button popped out, like a turkey timer indicating a well-done bird.

Since then, the navel seems to have lost its anchor and has never returned to its former shape. Now my little Buddha belly is starting to push the deflated turkey timer inside out. A small hood of skin partially covering the tip of the timer makes my navel resemble an old man's nose. I drew eyes and a mouth around it, which my two-year-old thought was pretty funny.

Because I have been mistaken for fat, my eating habits are concerning me a bit this week. I have already resorted to my former double breakfast and fattening snack in the late afternoon. This morning I had a large bowl of oatmeal and fruit, then went to Mc-

Donald's for an Egg McMuffin. I normally cringe at the thought of fast food what with so many nasty chemicals, by-products, and artificial fillers. However, at this point in my pregnancy, a drive by McDonald's sends my nostrils quivering into euphoric bliss with each whiff of grease from the deep fryer.

I sometimes hear a small voice telling me, "Why not opt for a healthy lunch today? It would be so much better for the baby." But the craving voice always seems to win out. "Gimmie that pastry, bitch!"

To give the craving voice a little bit of credit, I do believe that my body tells me what the baby and I require nutritionally. So sometimes I get my protein from a Big Mac. I'll just have to watch it because of the other extras that come with that dose of protein.

In the afternoon, I had an Italian hero sandwich and then later consumed a chocolate éclair that was about as big as my size-eight shoe. Mmmmmm, mmmmmm!

I frequently find myself wondering, What can I eat next? This could be dangerous territory! It's liberating to eat a lot and not be concerned about my waistline, but I have to remember that eating for two doesn't mean eating twice as much as normal. It means eating nutritiously so both of us can be healthy.

10

Week Twelve, Four Months Pregnant or Three?

Symptoms: greasy hair, headaches, nasal congestion

Although my skin seems to be clearing up (please let it continue!), my scalp is getting oilier than ever. If I do not keep up with daily washing, my scalp gets extremely greasy and itchy, and my hair takes on a not-so-attractive plastered-to-the-head appearance.

Along with the greasy scalp and zitty complexion, I still have the usual headaches—which are now getting worse due to added nasal congestion. My nose frequently feels stuffy, as if on the cusp of a cold. During the evening it is at its worst, as it is with all colds and flus, I guess. It's quite common for pregnant women to experience swollen and irritated mucous membranes at this stage of the pregnancy. Some even experience it throughout. My friend Carla had a stuffy, runny, and bloody nose from week ten of her first pregnancy all the way to the end. The poor dear never left home without a pack of tissues.

I officially have twelve weeks under my (tightening) belt: three months. Does this mean that I am now three months pregnant, because I have completed the twelve weeks, or am I into my fourth month and able to claim that I am four months pregnant?

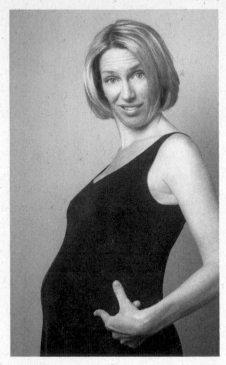

This has always been a puzzle to me. I must admit that during my last pregnancy I claimed being six months pregnant on day one of my sixth month. After all, I was into the sixth month and therefore that much pregnant. Right?

This theory works well for the self-esteem, especially during the last trimester, when other women are comparing their relative sizes to yours—when they were "that much" pregnant. The only time it becomes a problem is when you are in your tenth month and people are expecting you to give birth any minute. "Hey, when is that baby going to be born? You look like you are about to explode."

It is time to get creative with the existing wardrobe and make it stretch literally and figuratively. At this point, all of my pants are way too tight around the waist and fit only from the hips down. No, wait . . . I take that back. There is one pair of pants that does fit me properly—the almost obscenely low-cut suede pants that seem to be the fashion rage these days. I do look fairly ridiculous with my Buddha belly hanging out over the top of them, though. This is where the long, roomy sweaters and shirts come into play. I am pitching the clingy and going for the baggy. Besides, it's much more comfortable than the oh-so-fashionable body-hugging wear.

Back to the pants for a moment. If you have not discovered this trick already, here is a way to extend the wear of your existing pants before heading off to the maternity stores: Loop a rubber band through and around your buttonhole and then hook it onto the button of your jeans or pants. This way you can keep the waist semitogether with the fly partially opened. Be sure to wear something long and baggy enough to cover this fashion faux pas!

With my bod, it's also important to have a shirt loose enough not to show the girth of my middle, which does not yet resemble a baby in the making. It looks as if my adolescent boy body (remember, no hips) has swallowed a large cantaloupe or a small watermelon that is residing just about belly button level. When I look down upon my midsection in the shower, I can no longer see the top of my pubic hair unless I lean way over.

I suspect, if it is your first pregnancy, your belly probably isn't as distended as mine yet. Is it? Don't worry. It won't be long before you join the ranks of Buddha bellies!

If you are one of those unbelievably lucky women who have a perfect, compact little pregnant belly, then by all means show it off! Wear clingy sweaters, wear fitted tops, wear Lycra, damn it!

11

Week Thirteen, I'm Pregnant, You Know

Symptoms: headaches, nipple cheese

The headaches persist and have been most troublesome over the past few days. I had to resort to my prescription medication this past weekend because Tylenol was having zero effect. It seems there is nothing more physically draining than a never-ending headache.

Today I noticed that my right nipple is producing a bit of a cheesy substance, but not the left (yet). This time around, the changing state of my nipples does not surprise me.

Dr. Miriam Greene says: You might not experience these types of symptoms this early. Every pregnancy is so different.

During my last pregnancy, I was alarmed when I first noticed my mammaries transforming. The nipples themselves cracked apart into lots of little sections that most resemble taste buds. What was this? Eczema? Mastitis? Skin cancer?

Upon closer inspection, the nonpregnant nipple seems to be of a smooth texture, quite like that of the rest of your skin. During pregnancy, the little "buds" that appear are milk ducts coming to a head. In between each milk duct you may get some cheesy, sebaceous buildup (nipple cheese).

Did you also know that milk can squirt out of each and every one of these ducts and that there can be anywhere from twenty to fifty ducts in each nipple? I didn't know that. I foolishly thought the milk would neatly come out of one hole. As to why my right nipple is not doing the same as the left, well, I just don't know. I am not concerned, though. I'm sure the right side will catch up soon enough.

In terms of counting the months, I have decided that I am going with the I am now four months pregnant idea, rather than the I am three months and one week. As a matter of fact, in the past few days I have claimed being four months several times and all with positive results.

"Oh, you look so thin," "You look wonderful," "Who could tell?" Personally, I have a complex about looking "too big" too soon. It did wonders for my ego! And, FYI, our egos do need frequent feeding, as hormones and a distorted body can lower one's feelings of self-worth. So treat yourself to an ego biscuit whenever you can!

Now that I am into my second trimester, we feel confident that this baby is a "keeper." We are out of the statistical "danger zone" and I am now able to comfortably tell everyone—the people at the bank, the supermarket, the mailman, the neighbors, the garbageman, and anyone else who cares to listen.

At the supermarket yesterday, a woman behind me in line was looking at my midsection. I blurted out, "I'm pregnant, you know." She actually had no idea and was just trying to determine what kind of material my sweater was made of.

I had my monthly visit with the obstetrician today. I weighed in five pounds heavier than my last visit, but, in my opinion, that's not really a fair weight. I was fully clothed. Don't the nurses realize it is crucial to be as light as possible? Why didn't she insist I get into the gown?

Well, besides being slightly irritated about the weight thing, everything seems to be progressing normally. I got to hear the baby's *whooooooo, whooooooo, whooooooo* sound with the Doppler monitor today. It's always such a thrill!

I have decided against the amniocentesis test and I am going to have just the blood work done for the prenatal screening. That will be done during the next visit. If that test comes back funky, I may consider the amnio.

> **Dr. Miriam Greene says:** Combining a nuchal translucency (NT) test (a sonogram that measures the thickness of the fold at the back of the baby's neck) with a blood test that screens for maternal serum alpha-fetoprotein (MSAFP) is a good way to determine if further tests, such as the amniocentesis, are necessary. However, I do recommend that all my patients over thirty-five have the amnio.

I figure, why put any unnecessary stress on myself by having the amnio. I am just thirty-five years old so my doctor isn't pushing for me to get the test, yet. At thirty-five, most doctors advise that you get the amnio because at that age, statistics show that chromosomal problems may increase.

Besides, a big needle plunging into my belly makes me extremely nervous. Other drawbacks (at least for me) are that it usually takes two to three weeks to get the test results back (how stressful!), and at that point (about five months pregnant), do I really want to consider abortion? Also, sometimes the test results indicate that something may be wrong when it is, in fact, not. I have heard many stories about false positives.

Everyone has different reasons for having the test done. Some people feel that it gives them peace of mind, which is great. My friend Ava had an amnio for both of her pregnancies and was actually looking forward to the test and the results. She also claimed that the needle didn't hurt more than any other common injection. Ava believes in taking all of the precautions that she can. It makes her sleep better at night.

I just have a feeling that everything is fine with this baby and there is no need to mess around. Or maybe I am just a big chicken.

The wicked cold that has been going around has finally caught up to me. I had forgotten how cold symptoms can become elevated when you are pregnant. Did you know it takes longer to get over a cold, or any sickness, for that matter, because your immune system is operating at a much slower rate? And because all of the mucous membranes are already swollen, the irritation of a cold makes it all that much more so.

I never realized how dependent I was on the common over-the-counter cold remedies. While pregnant, the relief options are so very limited—a vaporizer (piddly), Tylenol (so weak), some nasal sprays (short lasting), and Sudafed (only succeeds in making me drowsy). I want my drugs back!

Dr. Miriam Greene says: Every OB/GYN has a little difference of opinion on what medications are permitted during pregnancy. For cold symptoms I usually recommend Tylenol, Chlor-Trimeton, Sudafed, or Robitussen. If cold symptoms persist longer than a week, you should see your doctor, as antibiotics may be necessary.

I cannot breathe at night. I have to sleep sitting up. My nose is so clogged I have to try and breathe through my mouth, but every time I start to fall asleep, my mouth closes. I have tried every position and my mouth still closes every time.

One thing that has not diminished due to this cold, however, is my appetite. Although I can hardly taste the food, I am still craving it like mad. Ah, well, as the saying goes, feed a cold and starve a fever. Right? I think it's time to make the brownies!

12

Week Fourteen, Moles, Skin Tags, and Third Nipples

Symptoms: bleeding gums, headaches

I have only one new symptom to report this week: bleeding gums. While brushing, I noticed a bit of blood on my toothbrush and in the sink. I should have already made an appointment with my dentist for a cleaning and checkup, but I think now may not be a good time. Getting dental work done is messy and unpleasant enough without swollen and sensitive gums.

I don't remember if the tender gums last throughout the pregnancy or for only a short period. Will have to look that one up. If the bleeding does subside, I will consider a trip to the dentist. Apparently, women are more prone to tooth decay during pregnancy. It's a good idea to pay extra close attention to oral hygiene.

The headaches persist. Jamey says I am going through Tylenol like candy. I just can't help it. I'm desperate for some relief. I wake up every day with a headache and go to bed with one every night (needless to say, the sex life has been nil).

I truly hope this pattern does not continue. I don't want our relationship to be prematurely aged, sexually. Will we end up being one of those couples that have sex only a few times a year? Will he not be satisfied and seek it elsewhere? Will I resent his lack of patience and also seek it elsewhere? Stop it, stop it. It's only been a few weeks. I think I may be getting ahead of myself here.

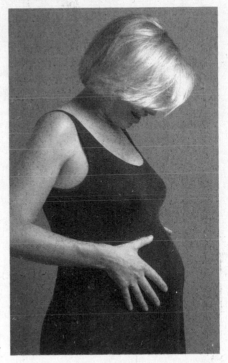

Pregnancy and childbirth definitely change a couple's sex life. Sex usually becomes less frequent, not as passionate, and defined by shorter sessions—mostly due to the fact that you are not feeling well, are too tired, don't have enough private time, and/or lose your desire. My friend Grace equated her loss of sexual desire to that of a former meat eater becoming a vegetarian. After you get used to not having it, you don't miss it.

There's also the other extreme. Nicole and her husband never had as much sex as when she was pregnant. Her hormones revved up her sex drive so that she wanted it all the time, which was fine with him. Unfortunately (for him), when the baby was born, Nicole's sex drive dropped to zero. As with all changes in a relationship (and pregnancy is a big one), I think maintaining a good sex life is just something you have to work at.

Beyond changes in the libido, more obvious changes can occur. Moles, skin tags, and third nipples are a few fun new things that can appear at this stage of the game. Although I am not experiencing many of these changes now, during my last pregnancy I did have some of these oddities.

My pre-existing moles puffed up to be a little larger and, in some cases, darker. Of course, seeing changes in a mole sets off the alarm bells for skin cancer. But, as I found out, it is quite normal during pregnancy.

Skin tags were something that I managed to miss out on, thankfully. Several of my girlfriends reported skin tags sprouting from their armpits, groins, eyelids, and necks during pregnancy. The unsightly tags can be darkly colored, like a beauty mark, or skin toned, and they usually hang onto the flesh seemingly by a thread. The only thing you can do about them is to have the tags removed postpregnancy—a minor procedure. Not quite as invasive as having a third nipple removed.

> **Dr. Miriam Greene says:** Most skin tags will disappear about four months after pregnancy or four months after breast-feeding has ceased. If not, it's a minor procedure to have them removed by your dermatologist.

What's a third nipple, you ask? Well, let me tell you the story of mine. I have always had an area of darkish skin under my left breast, near the bottom of my rib cage. I thought it was a scar from childhood (perhaps a chicken pox mark), and it always turned purple when I became cold.

I never paid it much mind until about the fourth month of my first pregnancy. It started to swell up like an engorged tick. I assumed that this fleshy colored nub protruding from my rib was a new mole.

After pregnancy and breast-feeding were over, I consulted a dermatologist regarding the still-existing tick-nub. I was told that it was nipple tissue and it had swollen as a result of the hormones released during pregnancy.

Most people never know they have nipple tissue existing in other areas unless they become pregnant. Apparently, it is fairly common (although I had never heard of such a thing!) for people to have excess nipple tissue within a vertical line of the breast from the clavicle to the hip. Weird, huh? Fortunately, my "third nipple," as I so named it, was not of the lactating kind and therefore was fairly simple to remove. I do have a small scar, though. Ah, well, just another battle wound of pregnancy!

13

Week Fifteen, Extra Padding

Symptoms: headaches, extra padding, bulging belly

I'm having headaches every day. I do seem to get a bit of respite about midday for a few hours. I hope this headache phase will be coming to an end soon. It seems as if I get phases of pregnancy symptoms that stick around for a few weeks and then disappear. When one phase is over, another one usually takes its place. Maybe the next phase will be the highly energetic, glowing skin, and feeling great phase. We can only hope!

I've had quite a bad bout of diarrhea this past week. I am not sure if I have a stomach virus or if it is a result of my pregnancy. Every day I have at least one gut-wrenching episode. It usually hits after dinner, which is the biggest meal of my day. Maybe, at this point, my stomach can handle only small amounts of food at a time. As you probably already know, a growing baby, moving your innards around, can cause problems with digestion like gas, constipation, and diarrhea.

I've started to notice a little extra padding accumulating all over my body. It seems to be most noticeable (to me) in the pockets that appeared over my knees and on my lower back. Retention of extra fluids and all-over extra padding are normal side effects of pregnancy and (I guess) do serve some purpose. A mother's body does need to have extra water on reserve for two, and the padding helps with all of the clumsy bumps, bangs, and falls a shape-shifting body encounters. Thankfully, the padding usually disappears after the baby is born. I had to laugh at myself today when I tried on a new dress with a low-cut back. My puffy back fat was bulging out at every point where flesh and material met. Geesh! Now I have back fat.

Fat in other areas is becoming more evident. There is no hiding my baby-bulging belly any longer. It is most definitely noticeable now, especially in clingy clothing. Today I had several strangers ask me when the due date is. I guess I am over the borderline of looking fat versus looking pregnant. Whoo-hoo!

I am still struggling with my wardrobe. This week I've got to find the time to clean out my closet and put away the "thin" garments to make room for the larger clothes. I'm still not quite ready for the full-on maternity wear, though.

Here's another little tip I discovered to extend the use of leggings or stretch pants—wear them backward. Because there is extra material in the back for your butt, you can hike up the backside of the pants over your bulging belly. As time goes on, you may find that this little trick doesn't leave much room for an expanding tushie. You, like me, may need to go up another size.

14

Week Sixteen, Another Leap up in Cup Size

> **Symptoms:** larger breasts, breast
> veins, nipple changes, quickening,
> heightened body temperature

The flu has been going around and, of course, I've got it. I won't bore you with all of the gory details of my ailments, but as I've mentioned, it takes twice as long to conquer any illness during pregnancy.

I have three deadlines this week, two meetings, and two birthdays to shop for—none of which I can do from my sickbed. It's so frustrating and *boring* being ill! I can only imagine how difficult it would be for me to be on an extended bed rest for the pregnancy. My sister-in-law was on bed rest for three months when she was pregnant with twins and never complained. She says it was nice being waited on hand and foot, for once. And she knew that once the twins were born she was going to have no time for such luxuries.

My breasts have taken another leap up in cup size. I had to go into the second drawer of bras on reserve. I found that since my last pregnancy, I have a range of bra sizes from 34B to 38DD. If this is your first, be prepared to keep buying new bras every few months. Don't get rid of them after you have grown out of them. You will need to use them again when your breasts diminish in size after giving birth and when you are finished with breast-feeding. I am finding that the larger my breasts get, the more prominent the blue veins on them are becoming. I imagine larger veins are required to provide more circulation for milk production. Well, while my breasts are looking more and more road-mappish, at least they are getting perkier. No push-up bra required here!

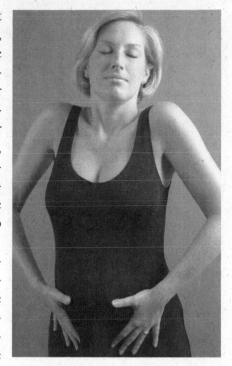

My nipples are also expanding in size and darkening in color—although the darkening is not as dramatic as with my first pregnancy. I think they still have retained some pigment from then. Most women's nipples usually don't return to their former color after pregnancy, but they may lighten up a bit.

I am starting to feel what is called quickening when the baby moves around.

Dr. Miriam Greene says: Most women begin to feel fetal movement between eighteen and twenty-two weeks. In a second pregnancy, if the woman is on the leaner side, or if the baby is very active, quickening can be felt on the earlier side.

I first felt it while lying quietly on the couch last night. I was reading one of my numerous everything-you-need-to-know-about-pregnancy books when I thought I felt a small presence moving about. What was that? Maybe it was the broccoli? "And the statistics of women having a vaginal birth after a C-section, are . . ." There it is again. Not quite gas, is it?

The movements almost resembled a fluttering feeling, as if I had swallowed a small bird. But it's the baby I feel! Amazing. So small, but already making its presence known. My sister-in-law said her first feelings of quickening felt like someone eating at her bones. Maybe her feeling was much more dramatic because she was having twins. My quickening is usually most noticeable in the evenings, after dinner. I suppose the transfer of nutrients gives the baby a good burst of energy. Sometimes it is hard to decipher between gas and the baby's movements (especially with a first pregnancy). There certainly is a lot of gurgling going on down there!

I don't know about you, but I've been feeling very hot at night. No, I don't mean sexy, I mean really warm. Apparently, it is normal for a woman's body temperature to be elevated during pregnancy. You are carrying around not only several extra pounds but also a little person that is a heat source on its own.

My body thermostat seems to be most elevated in the evening, during sleep. Jamey used to be the one throwing off the covers in the middle of the night, leaving me shivering. Well, the roles have definitely reversed. I can now sleep comfortably with nothing more than a sheet, while he requires the sheet, two blankets, and a comforter. I'm thinking we may need to resort to separate covers. We have been experiencing many nasty little fits of tugging and throwing of the linens.

I had another doctor's appointment this week and, thankfully, all went well. I got to hear the *whoooo, whoooo, whoooo* of the baby with the Doppler monitor again. At times like these I still find myself amazed. Hey! There's really a baby in there!

I had some questions for my doctor about my current navel situation—it has been very tender to the touch and protruding quite a bit. Because I always like to be in the know when it comes to changes and/or oddities with my body, I read up on the possibilities of what my condition may be. I had guessed at a diagnosis of a herniated navel. Well, I was right. The doctor told me not to worry—the chances of a piece of my gut popping through the hole in the abdomen wall are pretty slim. And if it does happen, I should just push it back in with my finger. Doesn't that sound nasty? If it does become a problem I may have to have a minor procedure to have it fixed. Ah well, it's nothing compared to a C-section, I am sure.

Next, the doctor and I discussed my plan for a VBAC (vaginal birth after a cesarean, or C-section). At this point in the pregnancy, most doctors begin discussing what your birth plan may be. I wanted to try for a vaginal birth this time, as I've heard from many experienced friends that it can be so much better all around. My doctor told me certain conditions should be met to achieve the VBAC. First, I should try to not gain as much weight as in my last pregnancy. Less weight gain increases your chances for a smaller baby. I imagine a tiny baby is a lot easier to push out through an orange-sized hole than an almost nine-pounder like my first baby was. Second, if the baby is correctly positioned and "drops" prior to labor, that gives my pelvis a chance to work on opening up. Third, if I go into labor on time, not ten days overdue (like last time), and have labor progress normally (without the aid of drugs, such as Pitocin), the chances of the former C-section scar opening are only about 1 to 2 percent. If labor is late and/or prolonged or assisted, the chances of the scar opening up go up to 3 to 7 percent. Sounds creepy, doesn't it? At that point, the doctor would recommend a C-section . . . and I would gladly have one.

Dr. Miriam Greene says: VBACs generally have a 75 percent failure rate because many of the same factors that prevented a vaginal birth may occur again. But if a woman had a cesarean section because the baby was breech or in fetal distress, she has a very good chance of achieving a VBAC.

15

Week Seventeen, I Am Such a Complainer!

Symptoms: headaches, hemorrhoids incontinence, shooting uterine pains

Headaches. Still! Almost every day I wake up to a searing headache. Thankfully, the last three days have been headache-free. Could this be a reprieve? Some women never get headaches during pregnancy even though they may have been prone to them, while other unfortunates experience them for the very first time. My friend Sandra never had experienced a headache until about her sixth week of pregnancy, and now she still has them frequently. Maybe the hormones of pregnancy flipped on her headache switch. She has been looking for that blasted Off switch ever since.

As well as fueling frequent headaches, the progesterone poisoning of pregnancy is aggravating my complexion again. I thought that I was over that phase. Ah, well. Welcome back to puberty!

Dr. Miriam Greene says: It's actually not progesterone poisoning. The flux of hormones experienced during pregnancy can cause a variety of disruptions in a woman's body.

If that's not bad enough, the hemorrhoids are back . . . and are already bleeding. The frequent diarrhea I have been having certainly isn't helping matters, I'm sure.

For me, bleeding hemorrhoids are par for the course. You may want to consult your doctor the first time you notice blood, just to make sure it's from your anus and not the vagina.

I am also starting to feel random shooting pains in my uterus. It usually strikes when I cough or make sudden movements involving muscles in the abdomen. I'm sure this is normal, as I experienced it before. During my first pregnancy, I remember getting quite panicked when first feeling the sudden, stabbing pain. What could this be? Premature labor? Today I'm not panicking, but it can be extremely alarming to others to see a pregnant woman suddenly grabbing at her belly and gasping.

The grab and gasp is the typical pregnancy soap opera move that creates immediate and grave concern for mother and child. On television, these tragic pains usually mean the end of a pregnancy or something equally horrid. In real life, it is just a usual, everyday occurrence and something to be tolerated along with the myriad of other changes that happen to the body.

Today, while away from home, I had quite a few coughing episodes (a leftover from my previous flu), and I found that every time I coughed, a small amount of urine escaped. I felt my underpants becoming wetter and wetter and was starting to get worried about the urine soaking through to my pants and showing. Will a wet stain show on black? Oh, gawd! Where is that sweater to tie around my waist? No, that won't work. I cannot tie *anything* around this bulging belly. Try as I might to have an empty bladder when I go out, it seems as if I almost always have to make a mad dash home. I suppose I could try to drink less, but then again, I don't want to become dehydrated. It's a losing battle. I guess the only thing I can do is to get going on those Kegel exercises to strengthen my staying power. They really do help, if you can remember to do them regularly. Pee, stop. Pee, stop. Pee, stop. Pee. Ahhhhhhh.

Dr. Miriam Greene says: I recommend doing Kegel exercises throughout the day, while sitting, standing, or walking. Do five squeezes per hour, five hours a day, and hold each squeeze for the count of five.

For the most part, all of my bodily problems and discomforts are related to this pregnancy. I'm such a complainer, aren't I?

I know, I know. It sounds as if I have quite a few complaints to report this week. Well, as I warned you, pregnancy isn't always a bowl of cherries. Some weeks, my list of symptoms seems to consume me. But, hey, if I can't share it with you, my fellow pregnant pal, then who? After all, girlfriends need to commiserate. I believe it is extremely useful therapy to know that you are not the only one with a hemorrhoid the size of a cherry, or having such wild mood swings that you contemplate divorce daily. When girlfriends really talk, they share the good and the bad. And it's usually the bad we like to air to our friends. If you have a really close girlfriend, you probably know more negative aspects of her relationship than you do the positive. Am I right?

Of course I do not complain to every person I come in contact with every day—only those people who are very close to me and who are genuinely interested in what I am going through (like you, my friend!).

I'm sure the woman at the bank doesn't really want to know that my diarrhea is aggravating my hemorrhoids when she asks me how I am feeling today. I reply, with a hand on my belly and a smile, "Just fine." She instantly brightens up and I can tell that she is genuinely excited about this baby, which makes me excited.

Smiles, happiness, and excitement are contagious. Even if you fake it, it could come right back at you and you'll catch it too!

One more note on complaining. In terms of husbands, you may notice that I bitch a fair bit about mine, but most girlfriends agree that your spouse is never more annoying than when you're pregnant. After all, his life is hardly affected by the pregnancy. He doesn't have to give up alcohol, sushi, and skiing. He doesn't have to suffer through morning sickness, hemorrhoids, backache, and fatigue. You may find yourself hating your partner. Don't worry. This is perfectly normal! Try asking yourself, Would I react this way if I were not pregnant? If the answer is no, you may be experiencing jealousy of his nonaltered life or just be in the grips of pregnancy horror-mones.

This week my doctor suggested that I schedule myself for the "big sonogram" at eighteen to twenty weeks. This, in my opinion, is the most fun test and the least uncomfortable. I will finally be able to see the baby and all of his parts. During the sonogram for Karmen, Jamey and I were so thrilled to see her sucking her thumb and moving her little legs around, almost as if she was doing a little dance for us. We should be able to tell the sex of the new baby from the sonogram, too—if he doesn't try to cover it up, that is. Don't ask me how I know it is a boy. I have a premonition about it, and I have been telling everyone that I know it is a boy. Boy, will I be embarrassed if it turns out to be a girl. (Not that I will really care if it is a girl. I already know that I love having a baby girl!)

Some people don't like to find out the sex of the baby before it is born, but not me. I am definitely a planner. During my first sonogram/pregnancy, the technician asked if I wanted to know the sex. "Yes, of course!" was my reply. Jamey, on the other hand, didn't want to know. I said, "Okay, I will just not tell you, then." Of course that didn't work out—he couldn't stand my knowing when he didn't.

16

Week Eighteen, Me, Me, Me, and My Pregnancy

Symptoms: back pain, expanding belly, leg cramps

A little more than occasional lower-back pain is becoming a problem. It must be the stretching of the muscles, ligaments, and tendons that is making me so sore. Well, I can certainly see why all of this stretching is going on. My front side is becoming bigger and bigger each day and I seem to be going through some kind of growth spurt. I would guesstimate my rounding belly to be about the size of a basketball—at least that's what it looks like I'm smuggling under my shirt.

I have some good news to report: I think the headache phase may be coming to an end! I have had only three this week, and my consumption of Tylenol is way down.

Being woken up in the middle of the night by indigestion or baby kicks is not yet a problem. It is the gripping leg cramps that are plaguing me. Last night I awoke to the pain of my calf muscle contracting into a baseball-sized knot. I could not unknot it without reaching down to yank up on my toes. The moment I released them, the cramp took hold again. Only after several minutes of massaging was I able to let go of my foot and lie back down. Of course, by then I was wide awake. I glared over at

Jamey's side of the bed as he snored away. Unfortunately, Jamey does not attend to my muscle spasms with a soothing massage like Carrie's husband did. My husband would rather not have his slumber disturbed. (Note: As I've mentioned before, you may find that there are 101 reasons to hate your husband during pregnancy.) It seemed Carrie's husband was always eager to help with any discomfort she had. He wanted to be there for every aspect of her pregnancy, from doctor's appointments to being physically involved with every symptom. Even when she got hemorrhoids, he wanted to examine them. That's where she drew the line. I think he secretly wished he were the one who was pregnant.

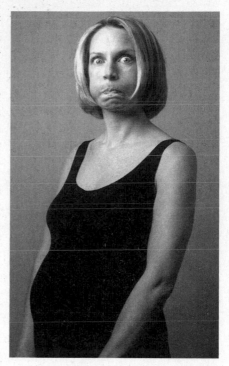

I've hit another milestone. I have finally broken down and worn maternity clothes. The options in my closet are limited at this point. All of the shirts have to be very loose, to accommodate the Buddha belly. My pants are not zipping at all anymore, even with the elastic band buttonhole helper. It is very uncomfortable, especially at the end of the day, to have a triangle of flesh gaping out of an open fly.

I took a trip this past weekend and had to put my bag into the overhead bin on the plane. I noticed the eyeballs bulge on the man in the adjacent seat when he saw that my sweater was not quite long enough to cover the zipper gap. I don't think he knew what kind of fashion deformity he was sighting.

That day convinced me there are times when maternity pants

would probably work better, even if they are a bit roomy. Donning of maternity wear is a big sign that I am definitely showing more. Sometimes it is hard to judge one's own body appearance—after all, you do see it every day and pregnancy is a slow progression. If she hasn't already, Karmen must notice that my shape is changing. Jamey and I have decided that now is the time to tell Karmen about her new sibling to come.

We put off the news as long as possible for a number of reasons. Two-year-olds have a short attention span and can get impatient. When told about an upcoming party we would be attending, she threw a fit because she wanted to go—and go right now. We also wanted to be well beyond the "danger period" and make sure this pregnancy is a definite keeper. In our opinion, nothing would be worse than to have to tell Karmen that her baby brother wasn't going to come after all.

Last night, we sat down on the couch and had "the talk." I'm not so sure that she gets it yet. I explained to her that I have a baby in my belly and it is going to come out in a few months. "This will be your new baby brother or sister." She keeps asking me to take the baby out now, because she wants to play with it. Karmen also finds it amusing to tell people that Mommy has "a baby in there."

While pointing to her own belly, she sometimes also adds that Karmen "has a baby in there" and Daddy "has a baby in there" too. Unfortunately, she does not yet understand that "a baby in there" also means that she should be more careful about pouncing on me. Yesterday morning, Karmen climbed up onto our bed and began squealing and bouncing up and down. Moments later, she surprised me with a full-on, elbow-to-the-gut body slam. Her eyes became as round as quarters when she saw the wince on my face. "Uh-oh, baby in there. Daddy's turn!" Two-year-olds do love to roughhouse.

Telling Karmen is about the only thing I can decide on lately. The decision-making chemicals in my brain seem to be all out of whack. Now, when it comes to making plans of any kind, I find myself asking someone else what he or she would like to do, as I quite often feel as if I cannot trust my own judgment. Usually, I am quite sure of what I want to do and when I want to do it, but these days I guess I am just not myself. There is one exception, however. When it comes to any decision based on food, I always have a definite opinion. I simply let the cravings steer the way. When trying to decide on a restaurant for dinner the other night, I had to call six different places before I could find a dessert menu to satisfy my need for a cream puff pastry. Not just any cream puff, mind you. My cream puff had to have the extra thick, extra decadent Bavarian cream filling, and lots of it.

Pastries are becoming a big part of my diet these days. A pastry or two are my usual for a late-afternoon snack.

Note to self. Watch those fatty foods. We don't want to become too large again, do we?

Maybe all of my sugar consumption has enticed the baby to be a bit more active this week. For the first time, I was surprised at lunch the other day by a real punch of a kick and let out an "Oh!" as if someone had hit me. A friend sitting next to me at the table leaned over and asked if I was all right. I brushed it off with a "Sure, fine," as I did not want to interrupt an intense story that was being told.

After all, it can't always be all about me, me, me, and my pregnancy, can it?

17

Week Nineteen, A Fight About a Fart

Symptoms: tightening under the ribs, flatulence, fetal movement

Lately, while driving or sitting in a fairly upright position, I'm feeling a tightening kind of pressure under my ribs. Reclining farther and arching my back is the only thing that relieves this discomfort. It is probably my shifting guts getting squished upward from the growth of the baby. Maybe once the belly starts to balloon more out in front, my ribs will not feel so compressed.

All of my gut shifting is also causing a problem with uncontrollable gas. Sometimes, when I least expect it, a fart just slips out without my permission! It happens most often at night. Last night, when Jamey got into bed, a foghornlike noise escaped from me. He was immediately angry and assumed that I did it on purpose. (Maybe it was because I couldn't stop laughing. It did seem quite comical to me!) He continued on his rant about my lack of consideration and rudeness. He was obviously looking to pick a fight.

Once I gained my composure, I was surprised and equally angry that he wanted to start a fight—over a fart. I explained to him (and he should already know, from experience) that passing gas during pregnancy is not always a controllable reflex. It had slipped out and I was sorry. That was not enough for him. He insisted that I did it on purpose and disputed the fact that it was a common symptom of pregnancy. The nerve! I told him to go look it up and get over it, or go sleep in the other room. I certainly wasn't going to take this abuse! Well, he finally quieted down and went to sleep. He never did look it up. I wonder if he still actually believes that it is not a common symptom of pregnancy.

While we are on the subject of not taking any flack, I should also mention that this too is another common symptom of pregnancy. Maybe it has something to do with hormones, but let me tell you, a pregnant woman is no one to mess with.

If you have never been aggressive or confrontational, you may surprise yourself with how much nerve you have these days. Not only does road rage take on a new intensity, but getting into an argument seems to be more of a desirable challenge, especially to win at all costs no matter who the opponent is.

My friend Sarah argued with her husband over the title of a movie for two weeks and insisted that she was right. Even after seeing a different title on a billboard, she maintained that she was right. She decided that whoever had put up the lettering must have made a mistake.

This week I am feeling a lot more fetal movement. At this point, the kicks and punches can be felt from the outside too. While sprawling out on the couch last night, I was slightly discomforted by the baby mambo. Jamey rested his hand on my belly and felt, for the first time, the life squirming inside me. His slow smile and shiny, wide eyes told me that this was the moment that the baby became real for him.

I had the "big sonogram" today—you know, the one test during pregnancy that you actually like having done. Jamey met me at the hospital at 1:15 and I was pleasantly surprised that he was on time (for once). There were no other appointments ahead of us, so we were whisked right into the technician's office and got started. I was grateful not to wait.

Unfortunately, having a full bladder is usually a requirement for the sonogram. It elevates the uterus and gives a better picture of the baby. Last time I had to pee so badly that I thought I was going have an accident as soon as the technician started pressing down on my abdomen.

After the technician squirted a blob of nicely warm jelly onto my belly, she began. (The jelly at my doctor's office was always cold.) The first thing I saw on the screen was the baby's rib cage and skull.

"There he is!" No matter how many times I get a sonogram I still am amazed that the baby actually is there. Also, to see the baby move, while feeling it simultaneously, is a wondrous thing. From what we could see, everything looked normal. All of the pertinent body parts and organs seemed to be in the right place and functioning well. While viewing the contours of the baby's face, we got to see him opening his mouth wide, as if to say, "Feed me!" (That reminded me I had not had lunch yet and was getting pretty hungry.) The baby moved his hands around and gave us a jerky little thumbs-up. "Everything is A-OK in here!" The technician panned down and we spotted the tiny legs and feet fluttering around. Craning my neck to see the screen was becoming increasingly uncomfortable, but I did not want to miss a thing—especially when it came time to see the sex. The baby kept moving his legs around, so it was difficult to spot the sex organs.

"I think I see it . . . I think she's a girl," said the technician as the X-ray-like images flashed before the screen. How could she tell? All I could see was a glowing blur of lines and shapes. She must be mistaken, because I just know it is a boy. After a bit more maneuvering, we got a better look at the sex organs, and I agreed that it did look like a girl—three little lines in a row, a tiny vagina. Where was the penis? Could it be hiding somewhere?

"Can we see that again?" I asked, as the technician moved on to the examination of the feet and toes. "I just want to be sure of the sex." Again, there it was—a little vagina. No penis.

A girl. I was surprised, disappointed, and excited all at the same time. Surprised and disappointed that I was wrong, because I thought we were having a boy. All of the predictions I have had all pointed to boy. (I didn't gain as much weight as last time, my belly was all out in front, all of my friends were betting on a boy, and the pregnancy just felt so different from the last time.) But I was also happy and excited because I know what a joy it is to have a precious little girl.

Most important for me, just knowing the sex makes the baby even more real. She is a real little person. She is my daughter and I cannot wait to meet her!

18

Week Twenty, Return of "The Buke"

Symptoms: bleeding gums, nosebleeds, Braxton Hicks contractions, heartburn

This morning I noticed that my toothbrush is becoming increasingly crimson after each brushing. The revival of bleeding gums and nosebleeds is common at this stage of the game. Thankfully, I was able to schedule a dentist appointment just last week, before my gums became all puffy and irritated again.

Because my mucous membranes are becoming softer and more swollen, it is no surprise to see a little blood in my tissue now and then when I blow my nose.

My friend Carla, who is also six months pregnant, has fairly frequent nosebleeds. Besides being pregnant, she's attributed one of the causes to be the dry, forced-air heat in her home. After putting a vaporizer on in her bedroom at night she found she was no longer waking up with a blood-speckled pillowcase. Moisture in the air does help.

After rinsing out my stained toothbrush, I set out and took a brisk walk with the dog. Hello—Braxton Hicks contractions are back! After rounding that first bend in the road, I felt the first pressure/cramp beginning. Amazingly, this was the same spot in the road it happened last time, during my first pregnancy. I remember thinking that I might not make it back to the house, that I could be in premature labor and might have to ask a neighbor to drive me to the ER.

Dr. Miriam Greene says: Some women experience Braxton Hicks contractions as early as twenty-four weeks. However, with a second pregnancy they may be felt even earlier. These contractions generally feel like a hollow, vague tightening of the uterus.

It felt like menstrual cramps, intensified and then spread out over my whole uterus. It reminded me of the crampy/nauseous/sweaty feeling one gets right before a bad bout of diarrhea. I had to stop and take a couple of quick, short breaths. After resting for a few minutes, the contractions stopped and I slowly walked home. I phoned the doctor and found out that they were, indeed, Braxton Hicks. Braxton Hicks contractions are quite common and normal for women in their third, and sometimes even second, trimester. Some women never get them at all. Marsha was thrilled finally to be experiencing what she thought to be Braxton Hicks contractions, when in fact she was in real labor. Surprise, surprise! They can be very uncomfortable, and even scary or exciting, especially if you cannot tell the difference between them and the real contractions.

Here are a few ways to tell if what you are experiencing is Braxton Hicks or a real contraction:

- The Braxton Hicks contractions are not as consistent and timely as real contractions. (The real ones are usually regular and increase in frequency and severity.)
- Braxton Hicks contractions (usually) do not accompany any other signs of labor (read about real signs of labor in Week 38).

- Real contractions (usually) begin in the lower back and spread to the lower abdomen while hardening the entire uterus. A Braxton Hicks does not completely harden the uterus—the fundus (usually) remains soft. To check if your fundus is soft, press down on the top of your uterus during the contraction. If it is not hard as a rock, it is most likely a Braxton Hicks.

Dr. Miriam Greene says: In some cases, a Braxton Hicks contraction may harden the fundus, but only for a short period of time, unlike a real contraction.

If you are at all concerned that you may be experiencing real labor, call your doctor and describe your symptoms.

Oh, one more thing—the real labor pains are definitely more painful than Braxton Hicks. But you wouldn't know that, of course, unless you have already experienced real labor.

Although annoying, uncomfortable, and distracting, Braxton Hicks contractions do have some use—they are rehearsing the pregnant uterus for real labor and delivery. So if Braxton Hicks are preparing the uterus for real labor, what is the heartburn preparing me for? Frequent vomiting during labor? (Some women do become nauseous and vomit.)

Why is it called heartburn? Is it because the feeling of scorching stomach acid starts at the heart level? I personally feel heartburn the most in my throat. Well, that feeling has returned, as in my last pregnancy. Every evening, about an hour after dinner, it begins. It starts with small belches and escalates into little vomit burps that land in my mouth. My friends and I have coined the term "buke," because it is a mixture of a burp and puke. (Pleasant, isn't it?)

Fortunately, my heartburn never progressed beyond the buke stage. My poor friend Michelle had to vomit a few times every

evening after dinner. Her
baby must have really been
squashing her stomach. I've
also heard that the progesterone released during pregnancy can relax the reflux
muscle that keeps all of the
nasty stomach juices down
where they belong.

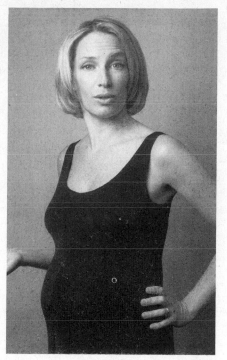

This is week twenty, so I
can congratulate myself on
being halfway there. I also
know that at this midway
point, most women feel
their best (during a pregnancy, that is). So I'd better
live it up! Now is the time
to get out to the movies, out
to dinner, exercise as much
as possible (if you're into that kind of thing), and maybe take a
vacation.

After eight months, things start to get pretty uncomfortable,
plus activities and travel are limited—not only by your doctor but
also by your own physical setbacks. Imagine going into labor
while out of town, or far worse, on a plane.

My food cravings are taking on a new level of intensity. Every
night after dinner I *must* have a bowl of chocolate or vanilla ice
cream, on alternate evenings. I never have been much of a dessert
eater, but during pregnancy, I feel I really *need* it.

However, I am trying to cut down on the quantity and frequency of my pig fests, as I'm concerned about all the pounds ice
cream can put on. And I now know that a heavy mommy makes
for a heavy baby, and one less likely to be delivered vaginally.

It seems to be very common with first pregnancies (at least
among my girlfriends) to go way overboard with the eating. Yes,

it is true that you do need to eat more, but letting the appetite monster completely loose from his cage can be diabolical. My friend Karen always had a problem with weight gain and consciously watched what she ate. When she became pregnant she let the appetite monster loose and gained more than eighty-five pounds! She realized how large she had become one evening while having sex with her husband. He had propped her up on the bathroom sink—and the sheer weight of her ripped the porcelain and metal piping right out of the wall.

I learned that I too put on a few at my monthly doctor's appointment this week. Last month I gained nothing, and this week I gained double the standard monthly average. My doctor told me I should "watch it."

What do you mean, "watch it"?! I thought. Didn't he look at my chart? I didn't gain a freaking ounce last month! Doesn't that allow me some extra leeway? I know I am still within the realm of an average weight gain for my time frame.

This time around, I am very sensitive to the issue of weight. Actually, come to think of it, I was sensitive the last time too. I think most pregnant women are. We know we should gain weight and at the same time we know we shouldn't gain too much so we get touchy if our weight is noted. We're pregnant, shouldn't weight be the last of our worries? There are exceptions like my friend Sharon, who couldn't wait to show and purposely put on extra weight.

My doctor also told me that my blood work and sonogram came back with good results, but he didn't elaborate on either. Was he purposely skimming over my chart, or was I overreacting? Was I just being sensitive and hormonal? When I left the doctor's office I proceeded to the nearest bakery to calm my horror-monal self.

While smashing the chocolate éclair into my pie hole, I couldn't help but drop some of the chocolate onto my lap (ooooops, I mean belly). The lap no longer becomes the target for dive-bombing bits of food. It's better to move the napkin out of the lap and onto the belly, because it will do you no good down there. Consequently, almost all of my former maternity clothes have stains on the belly.

When I became pregnant with Karmen, my friend Nicole generously lent me all of her maternity clothes. I remember thinking, Geesh, I never knew what a slob she was, because of all of the stains. Now I know better. Not only does the pregnant belly get in the way, but with loosening tendons and ligaments, utensils and small bits of food become hard to hold on to. Pregnant women are slobs. It cannot be helped.

19

Week Twenty-one, Cheeseburger Crotch and Flapjack Nipples

Symptoms: loss of bladder control, back pain, vaginal swelling

I have come to realize that I no longer have full control of my body. This vessel is most definitely a shared life-support system. The essential bodily function of bladder control has recently taken a leave of absence. While taking a walk yesterday, I was surprised by a sneeze. What was even more surprising was the gush of urine that escaped during that sneeze. I turned and headed for home as quickly as I could, before my wet underwear began to leak through my pants and show. A minute later, another sneeze put the squeeze on my already leaky bladder. I was soaked and could feel the warm pee spilling down my thighs and wetting my socks.

I suddenly felt seven years old again and out in the woods, far from home, playing with new friends and hearing the *squish, squish, squish* in my new white—but now slightly yellow—Keds. I couldn't let them see my wet shorts and sneakers. They would never play with me again.

Fortunately, this time I made it back to the house without being spotted in my wetted pants.

Another physical setback I have encountered is back trouble. I have been trying to maintain some form of exercise, but now it seems after every session my lower back becomes increasingly sore. My lower right back area, to be precise. I think that may be the sciatic nerve pinch thing that I have heard so much about.

Nicole had sciatic back pain for much of her first pregnancy, especially during her last trimester. When the baby was delivered, she said that her back hurt her more than anything. I can't imagine that your back would be more painful than your pelvic region during a vaginal delivery, but then again, I have no experience in that area . . . yet.

While exercising today, I felt the pain becoming increasingly sharp—as if someone was periodically stabbing a small knife into my lower back. When it began shooting down my right leg like lightning, I could no longer hide my wincing and sharp sucks of breath. I had to call it quits halfway through the workout. The baby demanded that I rest. Okay. Fine. I succumbed.

> **Dr. Miriam Greene says:** Temporary back pain during pregnancy can be normal as the baby applies pressure to certain nerves. Report sharp and persistent pain to your doctor, especially if it is accompanied by incontinence or if you're unable to sustain your own body weight. This kind of pain could indicate a slipped disk, which could happen due to shifting weight and strain put on the back during pregnancy.

This baby is becoming more active in her demands. I am feeling a lot of punchy movement at times when I am hungry, as if she's saying, "Hey, Mom! Get some food down here . . . pronto!" After a big meal she moves a great deal too. "Yeah. That was good! I think I will do a dance to show you my appreciation."

I am *really* pregnant now. There is no hiding it. Not even a baggy sweater can disguise the bump. Maternity pants are an absolute must and I can no longer stretch any of my regular clothes.

While most of my maternity pants are still too baggy, it is definitely better than suffering through an open-fly zipper scratching
at my belly on a pair of pants that can barely stay in place.

I'm also noticing that, yes, I'm really pregnant now, when attempting to get sexually intimate. The first thing that is quite no-
ticeably different is the appearance of your sex organs. The color
of the nipples and labia becomes increasing dark—sometimes to
the point of being purple, depending on your original skin tone.
Not only do they get darker, but they get bigger. Dime-sized nipples can expand to be the size of small flapjacks, believe it or not.
Also, your whole vaginal area seems to grow and puff up in size.

My girlfriend Grace said that it looked as if she was stashing a
cheeseburger in her panties, because her crotch had puffed up so
much. She occasionally asks me, "So how's your cheeseburger
coming along?"

Because the vagina is engorged with extra fluids and blood, it
is a lot more sensitive to the touch. This can be wonderful if you
have ever had a problem coming to orgasm during sex! It is still
wonderful for those women who have had easy orgasms—there
are more of them to have during pregnancy. Yahoo! This attribute
definitely goes on the pros side of my pregnancy pros and cons
list.

Believe it or not, during pregnancy an orgasm is no longer a
woman's secret because you cannot fake it. During and after an
orgasm, the uterus contracts and stays contracted for several
minutes. The large, loose bowl of jelly transforms into a tight,
hard, footballlike mass. It usually squashes downward and off to
one side. Don't worry; this momentary pregnancy deformity
doesn't harm the baby, although your partner may freak out over
the appearance of your belly.

20

Week Twenty-two, A Waddle

Symptoms: heartburn, bad skin, fatigue, waddling

I have had to give up my favorite pink lemonade due to my increasing heartburn, which has actually started interfering with my sleep—waking me a few times each night. Sometimes the Tums just aren't enough. Again, I am grateful not to have the experience Michelle did—heartburn elevating to the point of vomiting.

Last night I consumed several doses of Tums during my frequent bathroom trips and tried not to drink too much, as any liquid seems to make the heartburn worse. This morning I was greeted in the mirror by Inger Shimmofanning, a strange girl I knew from school who liked to lick erasers and suck on chalk. She frequently had a whitish-yellow rim of crusty chalk around her mouth that puckered the skin of her big, red lips. Inger and I were certainly no vision of loveliness. Where was the "glow of pregnancy"? I washed my face, brushed my teeth, applied some moisturizer and a little makeup. Okay. Now I should see the "glow."

I leaned a little closer to the mirror and saw the laugh lines deepening on either side of my mouth, the little red bumps of pimples about to erupt on my chin, the bags under my eyes, some broken blood vessels over my left eye and on the tip of my nose. Still no "glow." Personally, I have never been able to see the "glow" of pregnancy, at least not on myself. Ah, well . . . maybe it's the horror-mones that drop the ugly filter over one's own mirror.

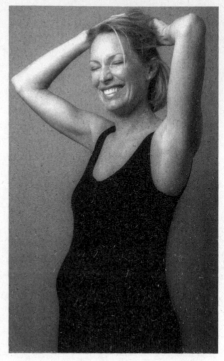

It seems that the fatigue is slowly returning. At about 4 P.M. every day I feel as if I desperately need a nap. Wouldn't you know it—my exhaustion kicks in right when Karmen gets up from *her* nap. I drag myself through the rest of the day and collapse on the couch directly after dinner. I wish I could go to bed at that point, but it is futile. That's when the bloating and stomach discomfort begin. It takes a few hours for my digestion to process before I feel comfortable enough to get to sleep.

During and after my last pregnancy my hemorrhoids escalated to such an extreme level that I had to have surgery. With this pregnancy, I am doing all I can to prevent that from ever happening again. The preventive measures I am taking include not straining while having a bowel movement; keeping my feet elevated as much as possible; sleeping on my left side; using Tucks, Preparation H, and other topical medicines; keeping bowels regular with stool softeners and/or fiber. Although my case was an exceptional one, do keep in mind that hemorrhoids are very common during pregnancy. The majority of my girlfriends have experienced them to varying degrees.

My friend Linda never knew what a hemorrhoid was until her twentieth week of pregnancy. While in the shower, she felt a bulbous and painful bit of flesh next to her anus. She screamed, called her husband into the bathroom, and insisted he inspect it immediately. Linda thought that the baby had dropped down into her bowels and was trying to push a fist out through her butt. Her husband loves to tell that hilarious tale after a few too many drinks.

I am feeling large these days. The weight shift throwing off my balance and my expanding girth have made daily mobility a little more troublesome. I notice my still-growing pregnant body the most when getting in and out of the car. First, I push open the door that now seems twice as heavy and another six inches farther than my grasp. Then I lean back and try to swing my leaden legs out of the door that is now about to swing back and crush my left ankle. I poke out an arm to stop the door and take a deep breath. Once both feet are planted firmly on the ground, I shimmy my fanny closer to the edge of the seat and slowly lift upward. Almost there . . .

If I do not rise slowly, I put myself at high risk for the soap-opera-style stabbing uterine pains. While making my tedious ascent I try to keep the grimace off my face and make my transition look as effortless as possible, as I know the prying eyes of strangers are everywhere.

In public, I also have to be aware that my weight shift and larger middle are affecting the way that I walk. I can't believe it— I am already starting to waddle! I caught myself doing it while walking down Main Street yesterday. It is true that it is more comfortable to waddle, especially in the later months. With a weight pressing down on an expanding pelvis and tendons and ligaments stretching, placing the legs farther apart is decidedly more comfortable. Sometimes you don't have a choice about placing your legs farther apart—thickening thighs can certainly increase that distance. Try walking with your legs an extra twelve inches apart. See? You have it—the waddle!

21

Week Twenty-three, A Different Kind of Wetting

Symptoms: heavy-feeling breasts, sores under breasts

It seems that my breasts suddenly are getting very heavy. By heavy I mean dense and leaden feeling. Sometimes, when bra-less, I feel as if my boobs may just drop off. Maybe the en-largement of milk ducts adds more weight than just your normal fatty breast tissue.

I'm not sure if it's the heavy breasts or the friction from my bra, but I have been getting small sores under each breast, where my brassiere rubs. The sores are slightly raised and red—not quite a pimple, not quite a patch of dry skin, not quite an irritated mole, but like a combination of the above. Needless to say, these little sores are irritating and make my bra feel like an instrument of medieval torture by the end of the day. The good news is that I do remember having these sores during the last pregnancy and I had them checked out. They proved to be just another symptom of pregnancy.

Carrie had the same sores under her breasts, on her belly, and in her groin area. Her husband refused to go near her until her doctor had confirmed that she did not have some contagious skin disease. Poor Carrie. At the time, she was extremely horny and had three weeks before her next doctor's appointment.

The bad news: I also remember that the sores, although small, did not go away until after I stopped breast-feeding. They must be hormonally connected. For me, this is yet another reason to cut the breast-feeding short.

When Karmen was born, I was prepared to breast-feed for at least three or four months if it went well (it doesn't always). I surpassed my goal, went to six months, and congratulated myself on a job well done. I thought six months seemed like a long time. Some women think it is abhorrent to deprive your children of breast milk for at least the first two years, while others never consider breast-feeding at all. In American culture today there seems to be no standard on the issue. As you probably already know, there are many pluses and minuses to weigh. It's all a matter of what suits you, your needs, your circumstances, and your baby.

My friend Marsha loved the experience of breast-feeding so much that she kept having baby after baby. She claimed that the feelings of empowerment, importance, and deep bonding with the baby were addictive. After five children, her husband finally put down his foot and said, "No more kids."

Dr. Miriam Greene says: I generally encourage breast-feeding, as breast-fed babies tend to be less asthmatic and have fewer illnesses. However, there are instances when formula better serves the baby—when a mother doesn't produce enough milk, is on medication, or is emotionally unable to cope with breast-feeding.

Hannah always knew she would breast-feed her baby. Her mother had breast-fed her three children and Hannah was more than happy to follow along in her mother's footsteps.

Linda breast-fed both of her girls until the age of two. She re-

searched and found many advantages of breast milk over formula; she was convinced that breast-feeding was best for her babies. It also gave her a little thrill to gall her mother, with whom
she had a rocky relationship, by whipping out her boob in public.
Once, while they were on the subway, Linda's daughter tugged on
Linda's sweater, saying, "Mommy. Titty." Linda pulled out her
breast and suddenly had a letdown so quick and so strong that it
shot across the car and hit a dozing man in the face. Whoops!
Maybe it was time to start using discretion about breast-feeding
in public.

I think I will try to breast-feed this new baby for at least three
months and see how it goes. Karmen's pediatrician suggested trying to breast-feed for the first few months, as it's an important
time in development and it can help build a baby's immunity. I
have heard that with the second child, sometimes breast-feeding
gets cut short. Maybe it is due to less time to spend with baby
number two, or maybe the mother loses interest. Is it less magical
the second time around? I wonder how I will feel. I wonder how
this new baby will take to breast-feeding. With Karmen, I was
lucky that she was a strong sucker but not too fierce.

My friend Clara's son sucked at her breasts so violently that
she felt physically assaulted during every feeding. She gave it up
when he cut his first tooth, at two months—her poor nipples had
become a bloody mess.

I also had a pretty good milk supply that flowed fairly effort-
lessly. A plentiful milk supply is usually a big plus, with the exception of the times when you lose control of your milk flow.
After the baby is born, it is almost impossible for a new mother to
control the leaking milk, and breast pads are essential equipment.
They are absorbent cone-shaped pads that fit inside your bra.
They are a wonderful modern convenience, if you can get them to
stay in place. After the birth of my first child, I inserted two breast
pads into my sports bra before a tennis game. When it came my
turn to serve, in a sweeping motion I dropped my right hand
down with the ball, and a breast pad came out from under my

right armpit, fell, and got snagged on the tip of my little finger. When I tossed the ball up, the pad went flying too. "Interference!" called the opposing team.

Breast pads come in handy because any mention or subconscious thought of the baby can unintentionally trigger the milk to flow. After some time, you can learn to mentally control your flow of milk. One evening, Jamey and I went out to dinner with a group of friends at a fairly formal restaurant. I wore a black, clingy top that showed every lump and ripple, so I decided to lose the breast pads for the evening. While still chatting, we all got up to leave. Someone mentioned the word "baby." Suddenly, milk was pouring out of my bra, down my belly, over my legs, filling my shoes, and then splashing onto the floor. In the dimly lit room, it looked as if I was peeing my pants. I made a quick dash to the ladies' room to stuff my bra with toilet paper—I didn't care about those lumps and ripples anymore.

22

Week Twenty-four, High Drama

Symptoms: back and hip pain, growing appetite, nesting

I've had occasional pain in my lower back and hip area that seems to come and go without warning almost every other day. Just yesterday, I awoke with soreness in my left hip flexor that became a shooting pain down to my foot every time I put weight on it.

I considered not going to work today but was surprised to find that I feel completely fine—no sign of soreness at all. Isn't that strange? Maybe the baby was in an awkward position yesterday, pushing on particular nerves that gave me pain. I guess that is how it is with pregnancy—some good days, some bad days. It certainly is difficult to plan ahead because I don't know how I am going to feel from one day to the next.

It's too bad that umbilical cord isn't also a direct communication line between the baby and me. "Hey, buster! Would you mind taking that foot off my sciatic nerve so that I can move, please?"

My appetite and my belly seem to be growing (again!) at an alarming rate. This baby could be going through a growth spurt. Believe it or not, I am craving sweets even more these days, and

we all know how detrimen-
tal those can be to your figure! I need to have a sweet
dessert after lunch and dinner. Maybe I should try
sticking to fruits to quell
my sugar cravings. Nah!
Who am I kidding. I need
chocolate!

Carla is also having a
hard time keeping her ap-
petite under control. She
claims to be hungry all of
the time (except after she
has just gorged, of course).
She even gets up in the middle of the night to fix herself
a sandwich because her
hunger pains are so bad. I

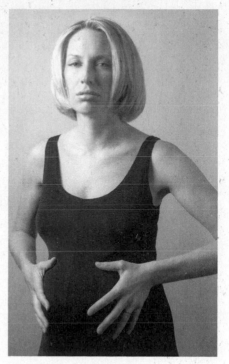

would rather suffer through the hunger pains than get my tired
butt up out of bed to eat.

I have started getting pedicures every few weeks, as I did with
my last pregnancy. I just hit the seven-month marker, and it's getting really difficult to get close enough to my toes to trim them,
let alone paint them. Imagine trying to tend to your toenails with
a beach ball attached to your belly button. Sounds impossible,
doesn't it? Anyway, this is the time to pamper myself, while I still
can. The next few months are only going to get more difficult and
uncomfortable. Now is the time to enjoy a few little pleasures.

I had my first fall (with many more to come, I'm sure) this
week. Toward the end of my last pregnancy I remember feeling so
top-heavy that I was literally toppling over every now and then.
This fall was nothing really serious. I slid on some loose gravel in
a public parking lot and fell to my knees. Although it smarted a
bit to skin my knee, I was fine. I was really more embarrassed

than anything. When I got up and continued on my quest for an afternoon snack, I saw that everyone within shouting distance had frozen in his or her tracks. What was I? Medusa or something? It took several minutes to convince everyone on the north side of town that I was "just fine" before I could escape into the bakery. I didn't know seeing a pregnant woman fall could create so much drama. Geeez!

I feel the time has come to get things in order and begin the "nesting" process. We will be moving Karmen out of the nursery and into her "big-girl room" within the next few weeks. I would like her to be settled and comfortable in a real bed well before the baby comes. We don't want her to feel that we are kicking her out on account of the baby. I'm sure we will have many little jealousy issues to deal with, so I'm trying to prepare her as much as possible. I took her to the furniture store yesterday to pick out her new big-girl bed. By her excitement, I could tell that she's already starting to feel like a big girl and big sister.

I also want to get the windows cleaned, have the trim on the house painted, get my garden planted, and do several other monumental jobs, including finally putting together a family photo album. As time goes on, I know my need to have everything "just perfect" for the baby's arrival will border on insanity. It's what nesting is all about. I kind of enjoy it, though—I really am such a planner!

My friend Bridget redecorated her entire house in only three months—during her last trimester. With the exception of sewing the drapes and building the furniture, she did it all on her own, too. She's what I call a "super-hyper-nester."

23

Week Twenty-five, Keeping
up Appearances

: **Symptoms:** heartburn, food cravings :

The only thing that is really bothering me this week is the heartburn. It usually starts at about 2 P.M. and lingers until the wee hours of the morning. I can't figure out what is causing it. I've tried eating bland foods, eating spicy foods, eating very little, eating a lot, eating only small snacks all day long, eating only big meals two times a day, eating lots of fiber, drinking only liquids, and drinking very little liquid.

Nothing works. Popping Tums every few hours does help keep the roiling stomach acids to a minimum during the day. But when I settle into bed each night, the heartburn gets well above "see" level. When I recline, waves of stomach acid flow into my mouth, and then back out again. It's not quite vomiting, but I can definitely taste the contents of my stomach.

Although my side of the bed has turned into a harem of pillows, it isn't feeling very luxurious. I need one pillow between my knees, one pillow under my belly, one pillow tucked beneath my lower back, and now I need three more to keep myself propped up enough to keep the stomach acids down.

The strange thing is that even though I have had real problems with heartburn this week, I am feverishly drawn to Mexican food. Salsa, guacamole, fajitas, burritos, tacos, jalapeño peppers, enchiladas . . . yum. What I would really love is a large, tangy, tequila-drenched, salt-rimmed margarita to go with my Mexican meal of the day!

One of the pluses of pregnancy is supposed to be strong, luxurious hair and nails. My hair and nails are definitely thicker and they are growing extremely fast. My nails have always been fairly strong, but now it seems they are a burden to keep at a reasonable length. My fingernails need to be short enough to have skin-on-keyboard contact for work. I've never been successful at stabbing the keys with a pointy, polished nail. My thumbnails have become as thick as quarters and I sometimes need Jamey's help to close the clipper. Watch out! Shrapnel flying!

My hair is growing at such a rate that it needs trimming and highlighting (yes, I highlight) twice as often. My roots are noticeable within weeks, whereas before I could go for many months without a touch-up.

To color or not to color is a question that has been debated over and over again. There are chemicals in the bleaches and dyes that may seep into your bloodstream during the coloring process. Do they harm the baby? Possibly yes. Possibly no.

> **Dr. Miriam Greene says:** Hair colorants and bleaches are much safer than they were just ten years ago. After twelve weeks, I think it's okay to color your hair. Note: During pregnancy, your body chemistry is different and the color may not "take" as well.

During my first pregnancy, I held off highlighting until my seventh month. I thought I would be able to abstain for the duration, but vanity and hormonal insanity got the better of me. Gaining too much weight and having bad skin, greasy hair, and dark roots was too much for me to bear. During this pregnancy, I decided early on that I was not going to put myself through that torture again and chose to highlight regularly. Trying to look your best does help with the sometimes plummeting self-esteem.

While we are on the subject of hair, I have found, through my experience as well as that of others, that it is best not to stray too far from your normal hair color or cut during pregnancy. It's easy to give in to a hormonal whim and just tell your stylist to "cut it all off."

Please, trust me on this: don't do it! There is nothing more tragic than a cute, perky haircut on a woman whose face is puffing and swelling with each succeeding month. By the third trimester, your head could end up looking like a pimple on a pomegranate.

24

Week Twenty-six, A Mosaic
of Motherhood

Symptoms: painful gas, herniated navel

Painful gas seems to be the flavor of the week. So far, it has struck me three times in seven days. As with the heartburn (which is now abating a bit, thankfully!), I cannot attribute my gaseous episodes to any particular habits.

While having brunch with my family, I suddenly felt a pressure rising in my belly. Even before I had a single bite to eat, my middle had swollen up painfully with rumbling gases. I didn't eat anything unusual that morning, wasn't overdue for my next meal, and didn't have any undue stress. I just can't figure it out.

Jamey was concerned that my gas pains could be premature labor. I explained to him that it was not contractions. Definitely not. It was more like the feeling one gets when eating five pounds of raw vegetables on an empty stomach. The sharp, bloating pains are soon followed by prediarrhea, pass-out-quality gas pains. When I explained it that way, he got it.

Excess gas is probably the closest thing a man will ever experience to having real labor pains. Sometimes I wonder if men can really comprehend and appreciate what a woman's body has to go through to bear a child. I know that I certainly couldn't fully comprehend it until I had Karmen.

I think this baby and I are beginning to develop an awareness of one another. There are times when she moves away from my spine and pushes way out, either to the left or the right, as if saying, "Here I am! Notice me!" Sure, she's noticeable, from the uncomfortable pressure of her propelling against my innards to the distorted look my belly takes on. Sometimes I can actually feel her individual body parts—her head, her rear end, and her feet or

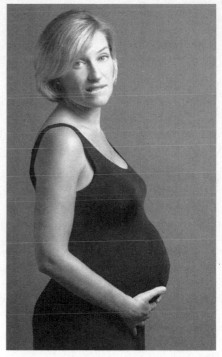

hands. If she's in a playful mood, wiggling her body and appendages around, I sometimes give her a little poke. She pokes back. We can go on for several minutes, jabbing at one another.

Too much movement can make me very uncomfortable (not to mention the fact that jumping on my bowels and bladder can release a fart and/or urine). Quite often, stroking her little body through my belly helps her relax and ease back into a more comfortable position.

My belly and I are getting along just fine, with the exception of my herniated navel. As I have mentioned before, I have a tear in the muscle wall under my navel. Once in a while guts or something pops out and I have to shove it back in with my finger. It's very unsightly, not to mention painful.

I have been told there is nothing that can be done to repair the hole until after the baby is born. Surgery would be useless while the belly is still expanding. So I guess I just have to deal for now.

After the baby is born I probably will have the procedure. Hey, I might as well have a plastic surgeon do a job on my stretch marks as well. I wonder if my stretch marks will get any worse from this pregnancy, or if the damage is already done. In my ninth month during my first pregnancy, I remember thinking that maybe I was not going to end up with my mother's saggy ol' scar belly after all. Well, I was wrong. On the ninth day past my due date, I saw the first shiny scar starting to radiate out from my navel. By the next morning the lone scar was accompanied by a gaggle of others, giving my belly that "cracked" appearance. Ah, well . . . again, chalk it up to the battle scars of motherhood.

My friend Marsha said she actually was happy to have "battle scars of pregnancy" and was delighted at the appearance of stretch marks streaking across her belly. As far as I know, there is nothing you can do to prevent these stretch marks. As with the sagging boobs, my theory is it's all due to heredity. There are also a number of factors that may or may not make you a candidate for a scar belly: the amount of weight you gain, heredity (the elasticity of the skin), how long you carry the baby, and possibly exposure to the sun.

There's a vast array of lotions, creams, and oils available to supposedly prevent the scarring. Although these topical solutions may relieve a little of the dryness and itching associated with an expanding girth, I can't say they will prevent stretch marks.

My friend Jennifer faithfully used a most expensive "miracle cream" from day one of her pregnancy and ended up with a scar belly nonetheless. She has got so many stretch marks it looks as if her belly was ceramic and has been smashed and haphazardly pieced back together again with purple glue—a mosaic of motherhood.

25

Week Twenty-seven, I Can't Decide

Symptoms: heartburn, leg cramps, heavy-feeling legs, emotional turmoil

Belelieve it or not, I am still having problems with heartburn, which I probably will be battling to the very end. A nurse friend of mine told me to try to limit my fluid intake at the end of the day. With fewer fluids in my stomach, I am less likely to have acid eruptions in my throat and mouth. It did help, but not without consequence.

I was easily able to fall asleep with only minor acid irritation but was painfully awakened by a muscle-knotting leg cramp. Yes, leg cramps again. I reached down, grasped my toes and yanked upward. The relief was momentary. The cramp took hold again with a new vengeance. Try as I might to pull my toes upward, they wouldn't budge. I gasped and grabbed at my calf muscle, trying to massage the cramp away. No luck. I had to get out of bed.

By this time Jamey was awake and grumbling, "What the hell's going on?" (He never is much for pleasantries in the middle of the night.)

I tried to ignore the gripping pain as I held onto my belly from either side and did a roll that brought me to the edge of the bed. As quickly as I could, I propelled myself off the bed. By this time, my leg was painfully distorted—the toes were all pointing straight down extreme ballerina style. I almost fell while trying to force my pointy foot flat onto the floor. Suddenly, it was over.

Apparently, one of the major causes of leg cramps during pregnancy is dehydration. I cannot decide which is worse—not being able to fall asleep because of heartburn or being woken up in the middle of the night with pain and distorted feet.

> **Dr. Miriam Greene says:** Leg cramps could also be brought on by a calcium deficiency. Make sure you're getting enough in your diet: about 1,500 mg per day—equivalent to a quart of milk.

My legs are also extremely achy. By the end of the day, my legs begin to feel heavy, and they hurt from the inside out as if there are large pieces of lead expanding in my lower appendages. I am not alarmed, because I know this is yet another common symptom. Excess fluids and weight can put a lot of pressure on the lower extremities and make them quite sore and heavy feeling. Although her doctor had warned her to stop eating like a heifer, my friend Karen put on more than eighty pounds when she was pregnant. I can only imagine how leaden and painful her legs must have felt in the later months!

When I'm finished with dinner, I usually prop my feet up on the couch for an hour or two while Jamey does the dishes. This, thankfully, helps relieve some of the pressure and pain.

Reminder: Use the "pregnancy card" as often as possible with your partner, especially if this is your first, and especially if there are certain chores that you've always hated. Be aware that the second time around does not seem to evoke as much sympathy and concern from your mate, as he now knows you can actually live through the pregnancy and delivery.

Though raging hormones are a consistent problem, I have been noticing a lot more internal emotional turmoil this week. I seem to be much more sensitive and irritable lately. The other day a friend of mine canceled a date at the last minute due to alleged babysitting problems. That's it! I am not calling her until she comes groveling! Bitch!

"Bitch," "whore," and "asshole" have become staples of my vocabulary, especially while driving. The slightest interruption to my destination by another driver sends me on a tirade of road rage and pregnancy-fueled profanity. Thank goodness people cannot hear the obscenities I shout within the privacy of my own car. A few minutes later, I usually look back on each incident with amazement at myself.

My friend Tammy once sprained her wrist while in the throes of pregnancy-induced road rage. Being from an expressive Italian family, she enjoys using strong hand gestures to get her point across. When a large red truck cut her off one day, she raised her hand and flipped her wrist around so quickly that she heard a snap. She, like me, was quite embarrassed at her behavior and could not bring herself to tell the doctor how she had injured herself.

Besides being sensitive, irritable, and angry, I am also often confused and am having difficulty making decisions. It is as if I have had the decision-making chip removed from my motherboard. At least it is comforting to know that I am not alone in this phenomenon—almost every pregnant woman experiences it to some degree.

I called up Carla this week to invite her to lunch. "Where do you want to go?" I asked.

"I don't know. Where do you want to go?"

"I can't decide."

"Me either. You decide. You are less pregnant than I am."

On and on it went. We finally let chance decide and flipped to a page in the phone book. I am fairly confident this decision-making chip will be returned after the baby is born. It came back the last time. Maybe the baby is borrowing it for the time being. Consequently, I have been relying on others to make the majority of decisions these days. At least that way, if all does not turn out well, I can blame someone else.

26

Week Twenty-eight,
"I Need Chocolate!"

> **Symptoms:** stuffy nose, ear popping,
> anxiety, depression, food cravings

This week I have been having problems with swollen nasal passages and ear popping. I'm not sure if this is attributed to the pregnancy or the spring allergy season (maybe a combo?). My nasal passages seem to give me the most trouble at night, while I'm trying to sleep. With one or both nostrils very stuffed, I tend to breathe fairly heavily at night to get enough air. Jamey has the nerve to complain that my "heavy breathing" keeps him up! He is the one who snores like a chain saw whenever he rolls onto his back (at least seven times a night!). With all of the swelling in my nasal passages, it is no wonder that I keep having ear-popping episodes as well. I find this to be most annoying while talking on the phone.

Yesterday, during a conference call at work, my right ear suddenly clogged up and I could not hear the client's comments. I had to switch over to the left ear and ask for a repeat (during which time I was pinching my nose and inhaling sharply—sometimes this breaks the sound barrier). It worked, and my right ear was operating once again. Seconds later, my left ear went out of commission. You can see how frustrating a simple phone call can be.

Along with frustration, I have been feeling a lot of anxiety and depression. I feel that I don't have any real reason to be depressed. I have been having frequent dreams of being chased, being late for something important, or witnessing a disturbing crime. Maybe the lingering feelings from my dreams are making my days seem so blue.

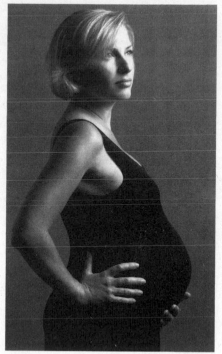

My friend Jane said she was depressed all through her last trimester and it escalated into postpartum depression (PPD) after the baby was born. Her doctor told her it was normal and is due to the major flux in hormones pregnant women can experience at any time. It is sometimes helpful to seek medical care and/or medication to cope with this hormonal imbalance. Jane might not have had full-blown PPD if her doctor had been informed of her depression earlier. (See Week 31 for more on postpartum depression.)

I have read that depression can be a symptom of pregnancy but did not (that I remember) experience it during my last. I hope this to be a short-lived symptom because it really is just so, well . . . depressing!

I am back to craving and consuming sweets much more often. (Not that I really ever took much of a break.) I have been to the Blue Duck Bakery five times this week. A little voice inside my head keeps telling me, "Watch it. This may get out of control." Depression says back, "Shut the hell up! I need chocolate!"

Each day it is harder and harder to find something decent to wear, something that doesn't make me look fat or too "cutesy pregnant." Is it too much to ask to have some stylish maternity clothes? They are extremely hard to come by and my wardrobe is in serious need of help. When I scour my closet, I feel as if I only have two types of outfits—pup tent or circus tent (circus tent being the one I wear for more festive occasions). If I could just find something that accentuated my still fairly thin areas—lower legs, arms, and neck—then I would be happy. I recently bought a few more maternity clothes online to accommodate my swelling shape. I am hoping they will look okay on me. It is so hard to tell by the pregnant models wearing the clothing—none of them appear to be more than six months pregnant. How is a person supposed to judge what a real pregnant woman will look like?

I had my monthly doctor's appointment this week, and to check for gestational diabetes I had to drink a sickeningly sweet glucose drink and have my blood drawn exactly one hour after consumption. I know it is important to have this test done, but I do have to complain about the drink. I chose the orange-flavored drink this time. I was told it tasted just like orange soda. I would say it tasted more like twelve cans of soda, but boiled and reduced down to one can of bubbly orange barf.

So I drank the sweet barf, got to the doctor's office on time, had the blood drawn, got a little faint, but felt relief that it was over. Now all I had to have done was the weight and belly check.

"Wait a minute," said nurse Carol. "Looks like you are due for another RhoGAM shot." "Oh no," I replied. "I already had one a few months ago." During my last pregnancy, I got one during the pregnancy and one after Karmen was born. With this pregnancy, I was given the shot early, because I had bleeding at six weeks and my doctor wanted to prevent my developing antibodies against my baby's blood, if it intermingled with mine. Guess what? The shot lasts only three months, so I had to have it again. What a pain in the ass! Literally.

27

Week Twenty-nine, Too Many Sams

: **Symptoms:** sciatic back pain :

I've had no new symptoms to add to my growing list this week, just recurrences and magnifications of some earlier ones. The sciatic back pain made a sudden appearance while I was walking down Main Street yesterday. I was carrying two shopping bags when the pain grabbed me and threw me off balance. To an observer it must have looked as if someone had suddenly dropped a bowling ball into the shopping bag in my right hand. It is so strange how this intense back pain can suddenly come and go. Sometimes it makes an appearance for only a minute or two, while other times it sets up residence and stays for days at a time. Nicole's husband was convinced that her random back pain was purely psychological—conveniently appearing when it came time to do the grocery shopping, the laundry, take out the garbage, or any other undesirable chore.

Another familiar condition has returned. Although I have been doing all I can to stave off the horrific hemorrhoids, they have cropped up again.

My friend Carla is also complaining of them now and claims

that she too has done nothing to warrant their arrival. Maybe hemorrhoids are just the standard at this point in the pregnancy.

The baby issue that seems to cause the most discussion is choosing a name. We know we're having a girl, so you would think that might narrow the field. Over the past several weeks I have been repeatedly asked, "What are you going to name the baby?" I find myself honestly answering, "I just don't know." Jamey and I cannot seem to agree on a name yet, but we do have several more weeks to decide. Right? I have already been through all of the baby names books and have not found them to be very helpful. I am hoping a good name will just come to me. During my last pregnancy, after finding out the baby was a girl, I decided on the name Devon. Jamey was dead set on Samantha—a name I disliked, mainly because I already knew of six other baby Samanthas born that same year. I was shocked and infuriated by how uncompromising Jamey was about naming the child. In fact, he was so stubborn that he told me no when I requested that we name her Devon while being wheeled into the OR for my emergency C-section. Can you believe the gall of that man?! After the baby was born, I agreed (under the duress of pain and mind-altering drugs) to name her Karmen—a name we both liked but was not a favorite.

Karmen turned out to be the perfect name for the baby, and we both grew to love it. Several days after Karmen's birth, I complained to Jamey that he had unfairly manipulated my decision by playing on my emotional and drugged state of mind.

On that day, December 6, 1999, he said, "If we have another girl, we will name her Devon." On February 12, 2002, when I had my "big sonogram," we found out that the next baby was indeed a girl! Upon leaving the hospital, I turned to Jamey with a Cheshire Cat grin on my face and said, "Well, Devon it is, then." He stopped in his tracks and exclaimed, "Oh, no. I never agreed to that!" This is just great! Now he chooses to have selective memory! We still have not resolved this argument. This could be grounds for divorce! I have never known any other couples to have so much trouble naming their child. Kathleen and Michael seem to have a nice system for naming their children—they take turns. Dan and Carla have agreed to name the children of the opposite sex. Dana and Max use alternating family names. I guess we, too, need a system.

Just between you and me, I think our "system" should be that whoever gives birth gets to choose the baby's name.

28

Week Thirty, The Propeller Move

Symptoms: heartburn, yeast infection

My poor, belabored bod has been through the ringer this week. My heartburn has become even more severe, keeping me awake for hours at a time. I'm sure my lack of sleep must have contributed to the fact that I have come down with another nasty cold, which has lowered my immune system, which has enabled me to get a yeast infection. On Friday night I battled heartburn for four hours. I tried to stave off scratching at my crotch for two hours, then had to concentrate on breathing for another two hours (my nose was so stuffed that I could breathe only through an open mouth and couldn't find a position that would keep my yapper agape). I had considered going downstairs to get the cork again when I finally nodded off (about one hour before I was due to get up).

I phoned my OB/GYN the next morning, pleading for solutions. Since I am now at thirty weeks and the baby is fairly well developed, I was allowed to take some stronger medications.

Dr. Miriam Greene says: For heartburn, Maalox or Mylanta is still the best. Small meals, throughout the day, also help keep it to a minimum.

For my heartburn, I now can take Mylanta. What a difference—this stuff actually works! For my cold symptoms I am able to take Sudafed Cold—doesn't quite do the trick but does provide some small degree of relief. For my yeast infection I am now using the Monistat three-day treatment, a messy but effective solution.

Since I have not been feeling too great this week, I seem to have a lot less tolerance for the groping hands of strangers. You know what I mean. It seems as if

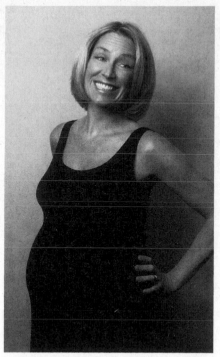

everyone wants to have a feel at you. It's not so bad when it's a family member or even a close friend, but a stranger? Come on. We pregnant women have to draw the line somewhere. After all, during pregnancy and childbirth, a woman's body gets more than enough touching, feeling, pushing, prodding, poking, and pricking from doctors, nurses, interns, and the like. The groping hands seem to be most common in supermarkets, while standing on the checkout line. A complete stranger will simultaneously ask me what my due date is and try to touch my belly. Sometimes the eyes of the random stranger will glaze over, as if he or she were a medium, waiting for the answer from a crystal ball. Once the hands are glued to the orb, it seems so awkward, if not rude, to push them off. I find it is best not to let the hands land there in the first place.

If I spy a strange hand darting toward the target of my tummy, I immediately spring into action with the "propeller move." I take my adjacent arm and swing it, in a clockwise direction, as if I am a prop plane about to take off. This very effective move was taught to me by my sister Kim. Although it does have the benefit of breaking the medium's concentration, it should be used very carefully. You don't want to be fracturing the arm of a ninety-year-old woman, or even hurting yourself. Kim once used the "propeller move" so quickly and forcefully that she sent a carton of eggs flying from the stranger's other hand across two registers before landing on the checkout girl's back.

29

Week Thirty-one, No Time for Regrets

: **Symptoms:** fetal hiccups, *linea nigra* **:**

Over the past several weeks I have felt a variety of sensations emanating from my womb—kicking, rolling, gurgling, stretching, and jabbing. This week, another odd sensation has started: the baby hiccups. This is yet another reminder that there is a real little person in there! I remember during my last pregnancy being puzzled and slightly alarmed when I first noticed my belly shaking rhythmically. What could this be? The baby's magnified heartbeat? Baby convulsions? Painless contractions? The feeling lasted for several minutes and then just stopped.

At my next doctor's appointment, I inquired about the new, strange feeling and found that it was the baby's hiccups. I thought that the hiccups were so severe that they had to be uncomfortable, if not painful, for the baby. The doctor assured me that it was perfectly normal and painless. Newborn babies also get severe hiccups quite often. I guess it is just a continuation of what has already started in the womb.

In addition to the growing size of my middle, I have noticed the telltale "dark line" appearing. It starts just under the navel and ends at the top of the pubic bone. The line, clinically referred to as *linea nigra*, seems to be a pretty good indicator of how ripe your melon may be. The more prominent and dark the line is, the closer you are to giving birth.

Women with darker skin tones tend to get a darker line. Almost every pregnant woman gets the *linea nigra* toward the end of pregnancy. Although I've never seen an "unmarked" ripe melon, there are a few exceptions among women with very pale skin.

I have heard that some Asian cultures believe the appearance of the *linea nigra* is a concentration of chi. The chi energy, creating the new life force, causes hyperpigmentation where it is most intense—the *linea nigra*.

During her last pregnancy, Carla's line was a very dark brown/purple streak, separating her melon into two distinct halves. She thought that her belly would always look as though it had been sliced down the middle and she would be banished from bikinis forever. That was not the case. It may seem impossible that such a permanent-looking mark could disappear from your skin, but the line does fade after the baby is born—usually enough to have your belly looking like its former self (if you don't count the sagginess and stretch marks, that is!).

The skin that is quite often changed by motherhood is on the nipples and labia. Although they will fade quite a bit from what they were during pregnancy, they will probably never be as light as they once were. Ah, well. Not such a bad thing for us pale-skinned gals. It's nice to have nipples that at least have some contrasting color to the rest of the breast.

Dr. Miriam Greene says: While this usually holds true for several years, a woman's nipples and labia will eventually return to their former color. On or around the time of menopause, they may get even lighter still.

I am starting to feel a little anxious over what changes in our family life this baby may bring. In the beginning there will be many sleepless nights, filled with feedings, diaper changes, and many hours in the rocking chair. Newborns have to be fed so frequently and the feedings take so long. By the time you are done feeding and burping, the baby has to have a diaper change. By the time you are done with that, the baby spits up. By the time you are done changing the baby into a new outfit, it is time to start preparing for another feeding.

I will become a housebound baby slave. I will have no social life. I will lose all feelings of self-worth. I will go insane with sleep deprivation. I may come to resent the baby. I do have some comfort in knowing what will be in store for me. I remember having some of these feelings just after my last child was born and I know how difficult it is to make lifestyle adjustments for a newborn. This time, I don't think I'll be devastated by the fact I am not an ecstatic new mother who can "do it all."

Most new mothers focus on how magical it will be to have a baby of their own to love and to hold, and never consider how the new addition may put a strain on their current lifestyles.

Clara was initially an ecstatic new mom, but after several weeks of sleep deprivation, altering hormones, and baby slavery, postpartum depression set in, big time. She became very distressed by the fact she was not able to live up to her preconceived "perfect mother" ideal.

Dr. Miriam Greene says: Postpartum depression is a very real symptom of pregnancy/postpregnancy and can be more extreme in some cases than others. Severe postpartum is fairly rare, affecting about 1 in 1,000 women. If your depression lasts more than two weeks and is accompanied by sleeplessness, lack of appetite, feelings of hopelessness/helplessness, suicidal urges, or violent feelings toward the baby, seek counseling immediately.

During many of our brief and interrupted conversations on the phone, she would ask me, "Why am I not in love with my baby? Sure I like him, but sometimes I just want to walk out that door and keep on going."

I tried to assure Clara that a certain degree of depression is perfectly normal. It takes some new moms several weeks to adjust— not just to the new lifestyle but also to the raging hormones that can alter a mother's mood. After a few months, things do get easier. The baby may be more set in a routine, enabling you to get some things done, and the hormones should be leveling out as well.

Now that I have made you aware of some of the difficulties you may have with your new baby, let me tell you about the good stuff.

I have to admit, I was one of those people who scoffed at all the women crowding around a baby stroller to ooh and aah at a newborn. Pullllllease! It's just a baby. And when a new mom or dad would whip out a wallet to display multiple baby pictures, I had to get somewhere fast. Booooooorrrring!

After the birth of Karmen, my whole outlook on babies was drastically altered. I was now right alongside the other women, drooling on the blanket of every newborn. What happened? I now saw babies as precious little morsels of life. I wanted to nibble on their snow-pea-sized toes and kiss their tiny rosebud lips—as if I could ingest some of that miracle into myself. I think the beginning of the lust for these luscious little creatures began only after I fell in love with my own baby.

I remember the first quiet time I had alone in the hospital with my newborn. What do I do now? I thought as I cradled her soft and warm little body in my arms. The baby felt like a loaf of baked bread. Then she turned her glassy brown eyes up to me.

Suddenly, like a blow to the head, I felt an emotion never known to me before. Was I going to cry? There was a spreading heat inside of me that was going to leak out all over the room. I felt good. I let it come and found that I could not stop looking at her and smiling. My cheeks were very sore that day.

The feelings of love you will come to have for this new little person will be miles beyond your current fantasy. The closest description I can give is to take the most passionate love of your life (you know, like that guy who made you sick to your stomach every night you were apart and put you on a pedestal of wild, woolly butterflies every moment together) and multiply that feeling by a gazillion. No, that still doesn't quite describe it. It is something that can be achieved only through experience. It's like standing outside of a huge cathedral with magnificent stained glass—you just can't see it from the outside.

Three weeks after the birth of her baby, my friend Ava asked me, "Why didn't you tell me how much love I would have for this baby? I used to think all of those goo-goo-goo-ga-ga-ga-ing mothers were just sickening, and now I am one of them!" I did try to tell her before her baby was born, but of course she could not comprehend it then. Ava and I now agree that you can literally spend hours just looking at, touching, and cooing at your precious little baby. It's the most rewarding entertainment on earth!

Just you wait and see. This goo-goo-goo-ga-ga-ga nonsense is really something to look forward to!

30

Week Thirty-two, The Divorce Is Off

Symptoms: heartburn, sore spot syndrome, Braxton Hicks contractions

The heartburn continues. I have awoken several times this week with a fire in my throat and a mouthful of vomit. Carla claims to be having the very same thing. We've been exchanging buke stories on a daily basis.

A strange new symptom started this week as well. I call it the sore spot syndrome. These tender spots on the uterus are usually localized to an area of about the size of an orange and remain for a few days at a time before moving on to another area. And when I have a Braxton Hicks contraction, the sore spot is the most painful area. If I didn't know better, I would swear there must be a large, purple bruise on that side of my belly. Maybe there's one on the inside. While visiting my doctor today, I was assured that the sore spots are normal. Sometimes the baby puts a lot of pressure on a certain area of the uterus, making it tender and sensitive, or the baby may push on certain nerve endings, which has the same effect.

The rest of my monthly appointment went well. Again, all seems to be progressing normally, with one small exception. The last few times I have been examined, the doctors have all noted that the baby is in the breech position. There is still plenty of time for her to flip, of course, but if she does not by the due date I may have to have her turned (if I plan on having a vaginal delivery, that is). Well, I'm not going to worry about the what-ifs just yet.

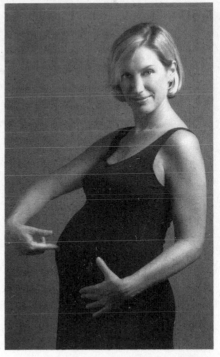

I am so relieved to report that Jamey and I have finally settled on a name. The divorce is off! The other day when I got home from work, a card from my baby girl to be was waiting for me on my dresser. It was signed, "Love, Devon Sloan": the first name I wanted and a middle name he wanted. What a pleasant surprise and a burden off my horror-monal brain. We have decided to tell friends and family that we still cannot agree on a name. Sure, it's nice to be able to share the baby's name with people, but there are drawbacks too. Some people will actually try to convince you to name the baby something else. Nicole's Aunt Edna was so upset with the name she and her husband chose for their baby girl that she threatened to leave them out of her will if they did not reconsider. Aunt Edna assumed that because the baby was not yet born, she still had a say in what the name should be.

I, for one, do not want the opinions and pressure of friends and family over a name. I believe the decision should be solely up to the parents of the baby. Period.

Another drawback is that if you tell the name, there is a chance that someone else may use it before you.

Helen and Barbara were the best of friends until they had the fight about the baby name. They were both due to have baby girls within a month of each other. Helen and her husband had decided to name their baby girl Samantha Jules.

When Barbara had her baby, a week before Helen, she named her baby Jules Samantha. Helen was furious. She could not name her baby the flip-flopped name of her best friend's baby. They had to start the baby-naming process all over again.

Unfortunately, Helen and Barbara never reconciled.

31

Week Thirty-three, The Same Three Questions

Symptoms: heartburn, leg cramps, frequent urination, disturbing dreams, headaches

I have had several consecutive nights of heartburn, leg cramps, hourly urination, disturbing dreams, and headaches. It's not fair that I am having sleep deprivation before the baby is born. I have six weeks to go, and if this trend continues I may be too pooped to care for the baby when she arrives. Some people say this is "nature's way" of letting your body become accustomed to sleep deprivation. I have a few choice words for Mother Nature that might rival my worst pregnancy-induced road rage.

I remember, after Karmen's birth, feeling a terrific sense of relief: relief from the burden of weight; relief from the constant pressure on all of my innards; relief from the heartburn and leg cramps; relief from the frequent kicking, rolling, and squirming; relief that it was just *me* now, and I could finally sleep! I'm not sure if it was the Demerol, the total exhaustion, or my huge sense of relief that made me sleep so well that first night.

My hospital bed felt like a haven of silky, white sheets, large, billowy pillows, and a mattress made to mold to my shape. It was days later that I noticed the scratchy plastic covering on the mattress and pillows. A tiny piece of blue plastic had actually pierced the pillowcase and made a small scratch on my cheek. (It's a good idea to bring your own pillows to the hospital. See Week Forty for a list of other must-haves for your hospital stay.)

I have realized that my pregnancy is no longer a private matter. There is no way to keep a low profile—I am an "eyeball magnet." Whether I am standing in line at the bank, strolling the supermarket aisles, or walking down the street, everyone has got to get a good look at what my maternal body has become. I guess it is just a normal reaction to do a double take or even to stare at something that is not an everyday occurrence. I wonder if this is what it feels like to be a celebrity, to have prying eyes watching my every move. Usually the longest and most searing stares come from a distance, where the stranger can most comfortably dissect my bulging belly.

While waiting for my usual toasted everything bagel with cream cheese, lettuce, and tomato, I felt a pair of bulging eyes on my left, boring holes into my belly. Across the sandwich shop was a woman of about my age, staring at me. Her eyes momentarily widened when she noticed me looking back at her. Then she seemed to soften as she tilted her head slightly and smiled at me in an admiring way. Her eyes said, "Good for you—you're having a baby. I send you luck and well wishes."

I much prefer the distant well-wishing strangers to the adjacent ones. While trapped in line at the supermarket, I frequently find myself answering the same three questions: When is your baby due? Do you know if it is a boy or a girl? How are you feeling?

I know these people mean well, but can you imagine how tiring it is to answer these same three questions twenty times a day? Do you think it would be rude to have a T-shirt made that says, "July 7. It's a girl. I'm fine, dammit."?

32

Week Thirty-four, The To-Do List

Symptoms: shortness of breath, puffy legs, cocktail weiner toes, nesting

During the last few weeks, my shortness-of-breath spells have been increasing. It usually happens after climbing a flight of stairs or walking briskly and is now being accompanied by light-headedness as well. Yesterday, after climbing the stairs at a regular pace, I was so light-headed that I had to flop down on a chair and put my head between my legs (not an easy feat at this stage) for several minutes before the sparkly stars flew away.

The reason women experience shortness of breath and light-headedness during pregnancy is that the baby pushes outward and upward, not leaving much room for your lungs to function. With a shortness of oxygen already, carrying the extra weight puts even more strain on the pregnant bod. I find it strange that I don't huff and puff during a heated bout of tennis. I am still able to hit that overhead smash at the net and then run back for the lob, over and over again, all without getting all wobbly and light-headed. I wonder if it's psychological or if the adrenaline rush I get while exercising enables my lungs to work harder. Hmmmmmm.

I also am starting to get puffy legs and feet. In the evenings it is most troublesome, as my toes turn into cocktail wieners and the

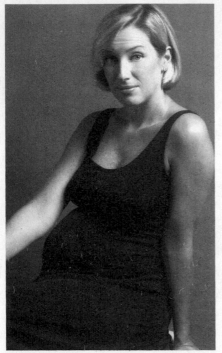

bones of my ankles disappear. The dull throbbing in my legs and feet starts to get me very cranky. I find myself leaving the dinner table sooner and sooner each evening, to put my feet up on the couch.

This baby will be here soon (sooner, I hope, than later), and I still have a gazillion things to get done before she is born. I have to finish setting up the nursery, wash and organize all of her baby clothes, finish my existing projects at work, finish the pictures-in-the-photo-album project, make a list of all the things I need to bring to the hospital, go to the hospital and do the preadmitting, get Karmen squared away in her big-girl room, get Karmen potty trained, do all the birthday and anniversary gift shopping for the next few months, and remember just what else it is that I have to do. This must be the beginning of the real nesting stage. Most women go through a frenzied cleaning and organizing spree just a few days before the baby is born.

My friend Tammy was on her hands and knees for eight hours straight, cleaning the greasy dirt that had accumulated under the baseboards of the deli she and her husband owned. Every time a customer entered the shop, her husband got the third degree about having her do such hard physical labor in her maternal condition. He tried to explain that she insisted on doing the job because it had to be done her way and had to be done "right." The next day, she delivered her son Andrew.

My sister was pulling up tree stumps, in ninety-five-degree weather, the day before her son was born. Her astonished husband came home from work to find her in her bikini, drenched in sweat and dirt, with a six-foot pile of stumps for him to dispose of.

If you have one of those undesirable projects that really need to get done but you keep procrastinating, the nesting time is when it will get done, if ever. And believe it or not, at the time you will really take great pleasure in doing the task.

So strap on the goggles and rev up that chain saw. It's time to clear that two-acre lot!

33

Week Thirty-five, The Perfect Labor and Delivery Fantasy

Symptoms: lower-back pain, fatigue

Lower-back pain and fatigue are my regular companions at the end of each day. I think the extra weight is finally catching up with me. Yesterday was the first day that I realized I move more sluggishly and probably will for the rest of this pregnancy. Now is the time to catch up on the more sedentary tasks—paying the bills, writing thank-you notes, returning phone calls, and so on—anything that can be done with my feet way up in the air.

Now is also the time to cash in on the pregnancy card—it won't be valid for much longer. When I was eight months pregnant with Karmen, Jamey and I went to see *Cabaret* on Broadway. During the intermission I attempted to go to the ladies' room and the line was about a hundred people long. All it took was one small sigh, and I was instantly escorted to the nearest available stall by a swarm of women who selflessly gave up their spots in line.

The same evening, we tried to get a taxi among the crush of people outside the show. I was prepared to do the usual six- to eight-block walk to find a better spot, when I suddenly felt the arms of a stranger guiding me to a waiting cab. The snowy-haired man and his wife, who had snagged the first car, were seemingly ecstatic to give it up to us. Far be it from me to deny them such happiness!

My OB/GYN appointments are now every two weeks. At my appointment this past Thursday, I was happy to find that the baby is now in the downward position. That's one load off my mind. Having the baby in a breech position this far along could be a big strike against my plan of a vaginal delivery. If your baby hasn't turned at this point, don't panic. There is still plenty of time left. Karmen didn't turn until the actual day labor began.

Speaking of "plan," now is the time to discuss a "birthing plan" with your doctor—if you plan to have a plan, that is. Carrie and Marsha both entered the hospital with no birthing plan. Carrie spent the majority of her labor arguing with her doctor, while Marsha's childbirth progressed with a fairy-tale ease. I like to be as prepared as possible. In my opinion, it's better to contemplate all the what-ifs before do-or-die time.

Some doctors routinely have expectant parents fill out a birthing plan, while others will discuss a plan if a patient requests it. The plan is meant to combine the parents' wishes and preferences with what the doctor and hospital find acceptable, feasible, and practical. The goal is to bring the childbirth experience as close to possible to the parents' ideal while minimizing unrealistic expectations and avoiding conflict during labor and delivery.

Here are some questions that you may want to discuss for a birthing plan:

How far into your labor would you like to stay at home? Hannah wanted to stay at home until the last possible moment, as she thought being in the hospital would be more stressful. The antiseptic smell of hospitals made her sick to her stomach. Jane wanted to get to the hospital ASAP for fear of a too-quick delivery. She had a recurring nightmare of delivering the baby in the checkout line of the supermarket.

Will you be eating or drinking during active labor? Some doctors advise against eating or drinking once active labor has begun, as it could interfere with anesthesia and/or other medications if they are required. Other doctors recommend eating to gain strength for the grueling journey ahead. After all, who knows how long your labor may go on? I found eating to be out of the question once labor began. I had diarrhea, cramps, and nausea that more than staved off my appetite.

> **Dr. Miriam Greene says:** I think clear liquids and light foods are okay for a mother to ingest during the early stages of labor. Once active labor has begun, I advise against any kind of food or drink, but most women don't want it then anyway.

Will you be using a camera and/or video recorder? Some hospitals, including mine, do not allow the use of video cameras (I guess for fear of lawsuits). This fact doesn't upset me too much as I don't think I'll have any desire to view how swollen and messy my vagina will become.

Does your doctor recommend the use of a catheter? Most doctors today do not use a catheter unless you need to have an epidural or spinal block. And, if that is the case, who cares? You can't feel a thing down there anyway.

Will you be using any pain medications? If so, what kinds? Personally, I am all for accepting pain medication during labor and delivery. It's good to be able to relax and save your strength for the pushing stages. Some women get so physically exhausted during labor that they have no strength left to push the baby out.

Some of the drugs (Demerol, Nubain, Phenergan, Vistaril, and so on) can make you sleepy or groggy, which may be a good thing if you need to get some rest. But as with any drug, these can also have adverse effects like vomiting or creating feelings of excitability or anxiety. These depressant drugs can also have similar effects on the baby.

My all-time favorite pain medication is the epidural. What a wonderful invention! Within seconds, the body-traumatizing contractions fizzle into minor pressure cramps. The epidural can save you (and your partner) hours of physical and mental anguish. But if you are going to have the epidural, you have to face that big ol' needle in the spine. Right? The thought of how creepy and painful it would be is a big concern, not to mention the fear of possible paralysis. My fear of paralysis diminished quickly when I found that the chances of that actually happening were just about the same as a house falling from the sky and flattening me. One recent study on the subject showed no cases of paralysis in 500,000 births assisted with the epidural.

And the creepy and painful part was really not bad at all. Contractions, and getting relief from contractions, were the only thing that I could focus on during labor. Having a needle put into my spine seemed so trivial at the time. I didn't care if the needle had to be administered through my eyeball. I wanted it!

Every woman I know who has had the epidural cannot praise it enough and admits she would take the needle anywhere the doctor wanted to stick it. But it is a personal choice.

One more note on the epidural: If you do decide you want one, it should be one of the first things you tell the admitting nurse, so that preparations can get underway ASAP. If your labor is too far along or you are progressing too quickly, you may not be an epidural candidate.

Some women don't require or want any pain medication. My friends Tammy and Bridget delivered all seven (between them) of their babies without any medications at all. They both claim that they never needed or wanted them. I wish all of us could be that lucky!

What kind of fetal monitor will be used? Internal? External? Most doctors/hospitals use the external fetal monitor, which is strapped to your lower abdomen. The internal monitor, which attaches to the top of the baby's head, is sometimes used if the baby has to be monitored closely, or if the baby's heart rate does not read well on the external monitor.

Will you require the use of Pitocin (oxytocin)? Does your doctor routinely use it? Pitocin generally helps speed up the delivery process. It also intensifies contractions, which is not all that pleasant if you don't have any pain management backup.

Will you need an episiotomy? Some doctors routinely do an episiotomy, while others exercise methods to avoid one. For example, the massaging of the perineum during labor and delivery can help the skin to stretch more easily.

Did you know that in Europe only about 10 percent of women have episiotomies during childbirth? It's mainly due to the fact that they have a midwife or nurse massaging the perineum before the delivery. In the United States, about 90 percent of women had episiotomies in 1983. Fortunately, today that rate has dropped to about 20 percent. It's still more than Europe, though. Last boat for London leaving at 11 o'clock, ladies!

Will the doctor need to use a vacuum or forceps for delivery? I always thought that forceps looked like salad utensils.

Will you require a C-section? I wish I had been more versed in the procedure when I had mine. With first pregnancies, most women never really consider all of the what-ifs. When I was pregnant with Karmen, I wasn't prepared for the possibility of a C-section. I was, to a certain degree, living in the "perfect pregnancy and delivery" fantasy.

Dr. Miriam Greene says: Pregnancy and labor and delivery are two different things. You could have an extremely difficult and complicated pregnancy and then have a quick and easy labor and delivery, or vice versa.

I now believe it's better to be prepared with all the information possible, before having to be faced with a major surgery. The sooner you start thinking about the what-ifs, the more informed and prepared you will be for your big event.

As with the "gory details" of pregnancy, women are usually kept in the dark about the details of a cesarean section. Sure, I got a brief overview of the procedure from my doctors and numerous books, but no one ever told me what the experience was really like— physically and emotionally.

I had a cesarean section the first time because, after three and a half hours of pushing, the baby was not progressing and her heart rate was starting to distress. The doctor did not think the bones of my pelvis were going to open up enough to let the baby's head pass. (This could have been due to the fact that she did not "drop" prior to my labor.)

A cesarean? I wasn't supposed to have a cesarean. I did everything right, didn't I? I gave up alcohol, sushi, Brie, and water-skiing. I took extra vitamins and underwent numerous medical tortures. I even abstained from highlighting my hair (until the very end). Although I was upset about having my "perfect delivery" fantasy shattered, I consented to the surgery, as it seemed to be best for baby and me.

A lot of women believe that consenting to a cesarean is admitting failure. Please don't buy into this old-fashioned notion. A C-section is *not* a failure! In fact, it helps to remember the ultimate goal—the birth of a healthy baby. We're not in this for the pushing or pain meds!

My friend Danielle was used to being fully in control of her life, from organizing a dinner party to planning her weekly copulation schedule. A C-section was not in her plan and consenting to it made her feel completely defeated. Later, she found that the baby's head was positioned sideways in the birth canal and with each push his head was just getting more stuck. There was no way he could have been born without the assistance of surgery.

There are a number of factors that may or may not contribute to your birth outcome, including the width of your pelvis, how much weight you gain, the size of your baby, the position of your baby, the progression of labor, the doctor's willingness to "work with you" through a long labor, hospital procedure, and other factors. Some things you can control. Some you can't.

Once a C-section is under way, you will no longer be participating in the birth of the baby. It's all up to the doctor to pull the baby out.

I remember feeling like a surreal observer during my surgery. Under the drop curtain, beneath my chest, I could see the doctor's legs bracing against the floor and then felt one hard yank. The event was over and the baby popped out.

I couldn't have participated in the birth even if I wanted to. As I tried to reach out and touch the baby, I suddenly noticed that my arms were bound down to two wooden boards. Your arms are bound to keep them from flailing and interrupting the procedure. Flapping arms are sometimes a side effect of the spinal block and/or anesthesia.

You might not get to see the baby for more than a minute or two. I got to see Karmen's plump little body for less than a minute before they whisked her off to be cleaned up and examined. I was struck by how much the baby looked like my in-laws. She looked like their daughter. Not fair! Later, Karmen did grow to look very much like Jamey's mom. I constantly hear, "How does it feel to give birth to your mother-in-law?"

When you do get to finally see your little bundle, you may be a bit out of it. I remember feeling so drugged that I had to keep shaking my head and slapping myself to be coherent enough to focus on the face of my baby. With most cesareans, new mothers do require some form of pain medication. It is, after all, a major surgery. It sometimes takes days to find the balance between the pain meds and a coherent world. This, in my opinion, is one of the worst aspects of a cesarean birth.

Although it is not ideal to have a C-birth, you have to consider that we are lucky to have the option. Before the procedure became a regular practice, many women and infants died in childbirth or were maimed from complications. Modern medicine has increased our odds of having a safer birth and a healthier baby.

Twenty years ago, having a cesarean automatically meant that all succeeding births would be done the same way. Today's doctors have learned that this doesn't always have to be the case, nor is it always most beneficial. But if you do have a C the first time, your chances for having another do increase.

Dr. Miriam Greene says: About ten years ago, it was generally the norm for formerly sectioned moms to try for the VBAC. Since statistics are now showing a 75 percent VBAC failure rate, doctors and patients are rethinking the plan and scheduling a lot more second cesareans.

With her second pregnancy, my friend Karen automatically scheduled herself for another C-section. She said she liked having a "plan" and didn't want to endure another bout of painful labor, just for the chance that she may have a vaginal birth. Plus, with a cesarean, she would have a longer hospital stay, which meant more time away from her mother-in-law, who had just moved in.

I would rather go for the vaginal birth with my second baby. I know from experience that recovering from major abdominal surgery and caring for a newborn is hard work. Several mothers (of both a vaginal and a C-section birth) have told me that the vaginal is a much better option—less pain and for a shorter pe-

riod of time. Plus, I'm really curious (everyone says it's more sat-
isfying than crossing the finish line at the New York Marathon,
popping a welting zit, or passing a giant BM). It would be worth
it, for me, if it works out . . . I think.

Will your partner cut the umbilical cord? If he or she is the queasy
type, it is generally not recommended, especially if you have a cesarean. Things get a little bloody beyond that drop curtain.

Who will be present during the labor and delivery? My friend
Celia had her whole family, in-laws included, in the delivery
room. She claims the experience brought them all closer together.
I, for one, don't want my father-in-law to see my vagina turn inside out!

Do you want to hold the baby immediately after delivery? My
friend Ava was so anxious to hold her firstborn that she reached
down between her legs to grab the baby before the child was fully
out. Sounds like she's got the skills of a contortionist.

After my doctor and I discussed my birthing plan, I was ush-
ered to the scale and was unhappy to find that I had gained another five pounds in the last two weeks. The nurse told me that it
was probably mostly due to water weight gain (I mentioned my
repeated evenings with the cocktail wiener toes). I did forget
about the last month of pregnancy being the puffiest stage. My
friend Jane was so puffy that she said she felt like the Michelin
Man. She was tempted to pierce the skin on her hands, ankles,
and legs with a pin to get some relief from the blown-up feeling.

The good news about water weight gain is it usually goes away
as soon as the baby is born (as if someone actually did stick a pin
in you). Don't be surprised if you pee and sweat a lot. Then, all
you have to contend with is the still swollen uterus/belly area and
some excess fat.

Some women assume that after the baby is born their stomachs will instantly return to their former, flat selves. It's hardly the case, but there are some exceptions, and I hope you are one of them. I certainly wasn't. After Karmen was born, my stomach was a little smaller and most resembled a huge bowl of jelly stuffed into a pouch. It took several weeks before strangers stopped asking me, "When are you due?"

My friend Jen described her postbirth belly as "a road map of downtown DC." Not only was her stomach big, loose, and jelly-like, but it was riddled with large, purple, shiny, wormlike scars. Word to the wise: Don't bring your "skinny" jeans with you to wear home from the hospital.

34

Week Thirty-six, Practicing Monkey Maneuvers

> **Symptoms:** pins and needles, stab-
> bing vagina pains, klutziness

I have been experiencing many episodes of pins and needles in the feet and legs. Sometimes, I even get it in my hands. This sensation is usually caused by the baby putting pressure on certain veins, arteries, and/or nerves. I have found that the best way to remedy the situation is to change position. Sometimes this coaxes the baby to do so as well. The baby is also applying a lot of pressure to my cervix and bowels. Sometimes I get a sharp pressure/pain feeling deep within my vagina that most resembles the feeling one gets during a pap smear. I know this must be the baby pushing or punching at my cervix. "Ouch! Would you stop that please?"

There are other times when I feel like the baby may actually be closer to coming out of my butt than my vagina. Last night, the baby had hiccups that I could actually feel in my rectum!

I am starting to have real issues with klutziness. I am constantly dropping my toothbrush, my hairbrush, my pen, the phone, a fork, my keys, loose change, and many other small objects. It wouldn't be such an inconvenience if it weren't for the fact that it is physically so hard to bend over and pick up things.

This morning I dropped the cap to the toothpaste. It slipped through my fingers and then rolled under the small, wooden cabinet. I bent at the knees and gingerly squatted down while trying to reach my arm under the cabinet. I could feel the baby's bones pressing against my pelvis and ribs, crushing my bowels and lungs.

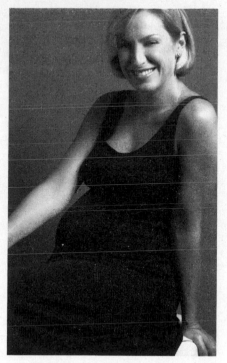

Some people think that being this big with pregnancy is very much like being overweight. I beg to differ. As opposed to a fatty stomach, my abdomen feels as if it is stuffed with a bag of rocks that does not give like a soft pillow of fat would.

The squashing of my lungs was making me light-headed, the pressure on my legs was beginning to feel as if my varicose veins might soon explode, and I still could not reach the damn cap! I slapped both hands on the cool floor, got on all fours, and let my head hang down. I took a couple of deep breaths before the sparkly stars began to clear from my vision. I lowered my face to peer under the cabinet and the sparkles returned. Before they completely obscured my vision, I jabbed a hand under the cabinet and snagged the cap. Victory! Now all I had to do was get up.

I know this klutzy period will probably continue to the end of the pregnancy. I guess I am going to start practicing my monkey maneuvers—picking up small objects with my toes.

The clumsy phase is mainly caused by the natural loosening and stretching of the tendons and ligaments during the last trimester. It is definitely harder to maintain a once taken-for-granted manual dexterity.

My friend Jane was so clumsy in her last month of pregnancy that she imagined she would be unable to hold her newborn, for fear of dropping her. Of course that didn't happen.

35

Week Thirty-seven, Crotch Conscientious

> **Symptoms:** frequent urination, saddle sore, hemorrhoids

The baby "dropped" this week, meaning her head has descended deep into my pelvis and she is in the birthing position. This also means a lot more discomfort for me. The pelvic pressure is putting a real squeeze on my bladder. It seems I can hold only about five ounces of fluid at a time. The weight of the baby must also be working on opening up the bones of my pelvis, as I now feel sore, as if I have been horseback riding for a solid week. The biggest problem this dropping has caused is—guess what?—the hemorrhoids. They are back again and worse than ever.

During the last trimester, it is very common for those chronic problems to flare up again. Nicole had the torn ligaments in her back act up again. Carla had her pulled groin injury return. Jill had her varicose veins throbbing, to the beat of her heart, once again.

With all the stress a woman's pregnant body goes through, I guess it's natural to have a bit of a breakdown near the end.

Well, the time is drawing close and I am now having a weekly visit to the doctor—to check for effacement, dilation, and so on.

These appointments, of course, include the weekly pelvic exam, which is more uncomfortable than ever. Since your vagina and cervix are so engorged and sensitive, the poking and prodding of an internal exam feels about as good as a massage on sore PMS boobs.

My friend Grace is visiting me this week. She's also pregnant and is just beginning her second trimester. She had no interest in accompanying me to my weekly appointment until I mentioned that we might be able to sneak out the Doppler and listen to her baby's heartbeat too. While we were waiting for the doctor, we spied the Doppler and lubricating jelly readied for use on the counter. Grace snatched up the tube of jelly so excitedly that she squeezed too hard and a big snake of it splattered on the floor.

"Ah, well. We'll get to that later," I said as I grabbed the Doppler, swabbed up some jelly and began rubbing it around on her belly. The machine gave a loud *crack* and we screamed and laughed. The volume had been left on the highest setting.

We finally did get it to work properly and we got to hear her baby's *whoooooo, whooooo, whooooo* noise. We were both so mesmerized that we didn't immediately notice the rustling of papers outside the door. The doctor was looking over my chart and about to enter. Ack!

Quick! Clean off the Doppler! Put it back in position! Put the cap back on the jelly!! In a slapstick, panicked fashion, we got everything into place just as the door began to open. Oooooops! We forgot the mess of jelly on the floor! Grace casually took off her shoe and wiped it up with her sock. Whew!

After my exam, I have to report there is still nothing going on. I guess the dropping of the baby has not done anything yet. Drat!

Since I am having my weekly pelvic exams and the baby could be born anytime, I am now a lot more concerned about how things are looking "down there." It's time to schedule myself for another bikini wax, although it is most painful this far along in the pregnancy. I would like to have my crotch as neat and clean as

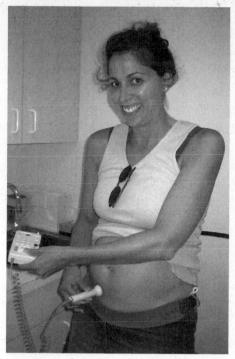

Sneaking a listen with the Doppler.

possible for all the viewing it is going to get. And I certainly cannot shave and/or trim my own pubic hair at this point. As you know, you cannot see a thing down there. It's quite a feat, even with the assistance of a mirror.

Last week I made an attempt at cleaning things up by using my husband's electric razor. I was hovering over the toilet, trying to shave by feel alone. I felt a little sting, brought the razor up from under my orb, and noticed a good amount of blood on the razor, dripping down to my hand. Oh geesh! I guess I cut myself pretty good. The room started to spin and I had to plop down on the toilet and drop my head to feel better. Needless to say, I did only a half-assed job.

I remember from my first pregnancy being quite concerned over the fact that many people were going to be staring at my crotch, possibly for hours, during the labor and delivery. I imagined being extremely humiliated and embarrassed. Well, I am happy to report that did not happen and has never happened to anyone I know. During labor in the hospital, with all of the nurses and doctors examining you, modesty will be the farthest thing from your mind. Maybe labor releases some kind of anti-inhibition chemical?

My to-do list before this baby is born is getting shorter. There is an end in sight. Maybe the baby will be born when I check my last item on that list. If that is the case, I'd better get cracking—I want this baby born sooner rather than later.

I have a feeling that I may go into labor next week, when the moon is full. I have been told that a full moon can be a catalyst for labor. It is also a proven fact that maternity wards are usually the most crowded during the full moon. Yippee!

36

Week Thirty-eight, I Want My Body Back!

Symptoms: stabbing back pain, Braxton Hicks contractions, heartburn, faintness, shortness of breath, nausea, fatigue

No new symptoms to report this week, only the return of previous issues. I have been having a dreadful combination of stabbing back pain, lots of Braxton Hicks contractions, plenty of heartburn, faintness, shortness of breath, and periods of nausea and fatigue.

I cannot find any position (sitting, standing, or lying down) that is not painful or bothersome. It would be more comfortable if the baby were out. Yes, did you hear that, baby? You can come out now!

I can honestly say that I have had it. I want my body back. No more sharing! I know the baby will be a lot more work once she is out in this world, but at this point, I'm willing to do it if I can get some relief from my many discomforts. In the evenings I find myself at my most uncomfortable and cranky.

Last night I overheard Jamey on the phone, saying that he wishes this baby would be born soon. He said he wants his wife back. I think this is a common wish among fathers-to-be. Then again, Linda's husband became more and more excited about his

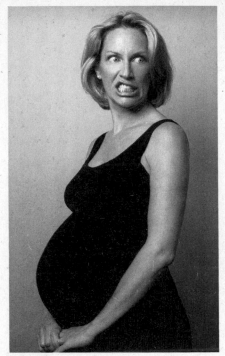

son's pending birth and seemed to enjoy every moment of the pregnancy. He must be the exception to the rule.

Only two more days until the full moon. That has got to be the date! I have been patiently looking for the signs of labor, or even prelabor. Every time I go to the bathroom, I check the toilet paper for the mucous plug. Nothing. Every time I get up out of bed, I expect my water to break. Nothing. Every time I have a Braxton Hicks contraction, I check the clock to see if it will progress to contractions at regular intervals. Nothing.

The signs of labor/prelabor can be different with every person, and even with every pregnancy. While we are waiting, here is a list of things to look for:

The baby drops. This usually happens two to four weeks before the onset of labor in first-time mothers. With second births and beyond, the dropping is said to be rare until the actual onset of real labor. Ha! Not for me. I feel as if I have been riding on this cattle drive for more than two weeks now. The fetus descends into the pelvis and usually creates feelings of more pressure in the pelvis, groin, and rectum.

The nesting frenzy. A spurt of energy accompanied by an uncontrollable urge to clean, arrange, or organize. This could happen weeks before real labor, or just hours before. Maybe I have already had my nesting frenzy. I no longer am having birdlike bursts of energy that enable me to check off more than twenty items a day.

The loss of the mucous plug. As the cervix begins to thin out and open, the cork of mucous that seals the opening drops out. You might see this thick glob in your underwear as early as two weeks before delivery, or just as labor begins. Karen was initially very angry with her husband when she lost her mucous plug. She thought he had missed the wastebasket and spit into the laundry. It turned out the blob in her underwear was not a loogie of his after all.

The "bloody show." As the cervix dilates, capillaries rupture, making vaginal discharge pink or streaked with blood. Again, this could be the beginning of real labor, or you may still be days away. I remember seeing blood on a wad of toilet paper as my contractions were beginning with Karmen. Disappointingly, my real labor didn't begin for another four days. Oh, bloody hell!

Diarrhea. Sometimes happens with the onset of labor. This may be nature's way of making sure you are "cleaned out" before the birth. Well, I have been experiencing diarrhea, randomly, for a week and have been feeling far from "clean" afterward.

Contractions intensify and become more frequent. The pain usually begins in the lower back and then spreads to the abdomen. Also, the contractions are not relieved by a change in position. (See Week 39 for what contractions really feel like.)

Membranes rupture/water breaks. In only about 15 percent of women the water breaks, in a gush or a trickle, before labor begins. If that is the case, real labor usually begins within a few hours of the rupture. Most doctors want the baby delivered within twenty-four hours to prevent possible infection and may induce labor if you are not progressing.

During my first pregnancy, my water broke on my third day of contractions/false labor. By this time, I had become a real expert on the breathing techniques used to get through the pain of contractions. I found the Lamaze technique of breathing during contractions to be the most helpful. The exercise of taking rhythmic breaths gives your body oxygen, helps distract your mind from pain, and makes you more relaxed. Lamaze breathing is the most useful thing I learned from any prenatal class.

> **Dr. Miriam Greene says:** There are a variety of birthing techniques that can help you through the discomforts of labor and delivery, including Lamaze, the Bradley method, water birthing, sensory distraction, and hypnosis. You can ask your doctor or local hospital for information on where to sign up for such classes.

Although I was managing the pain, I was exhausted from being kept awake for days. The rupturing of membranes was a welcome surprise.

I got out of bed and suddenly felt a warm gush between my legs. I immediately grabbed my crotch and got to the toilet. More gushes of water. So this was it! I was going to have the baby now. I got into the shower, blow-dried my hair, and put on a little makeup. In my opinion, it's good to be as clean as you can when you leave for the hospital. Who knows when you will be able to take another shower.

I had to cover the bathroom floor with many layers of towels to catch all of the water that was being expelled every time I had a contraction. It felt like gallons! All the while, my husband and father were screaming at me, "This baby is going to come any minute. Let's go. Let's go. Let's go!" I finally got dressed and went downstairs, with a towel in my underwear to catch any more water that might come.

As I was about to step out the door, another contraction came and filled the towel with water. It went down my legs, filled my shoes, and splashed onto the floor. I thought my father was going to faint from the horror of it (he is quite conservative and does not enjoy being witness to "womanly" things).

My friend Camilla, on the other hand, had the opposite extreme. Near the end of her pregnancy, her doctor had determined that her amniotic fluid had almost completely dried up. Her labor was induced, and she never had so much as a trickle of water.

Most first-time mothers fear the embarrassment of breaking water in a public place. I'm sure you must have heard the proverbial story of a woman carrying a jar of pickles with her through the supermarket, to drop just in case her water broke.

I hope you will take some small comfort in knowing that if you are among the very small percentage of women that it happens to in public, you will probably look back on it as no big deal—just like the fact that your crotch will be hanging out there, for hours, for many people to see. I promise you will get over it.

Although the jar of pickles can provide a good scapegoat, it is not always feasible. I do suggest having a few spare towels stashed in your car, though. If you happen to have as much fluid as I did, towels may help preserve the upholstery.

37

Week Thirty-nine, Not
Taking Any Shit

Symptoms: puffiness in legs and feet, back pain, Braxton Hicks contractions, heartburn, faintness, shortness of breath, nausea, fatigue, sore pelvis, throbbing feet

I can add one more thing to last week's list: more puffiness in my legs and feet. I have been trying to keep them elevated as much as possible, which does help . . . a little. This relentless combination of symptoms is making me quite cranky. My patience and temper have been extremely short during periods of maximum discomfort.

My current mind-set is: If you are not experiencing back pain, Braxton Hicks contractions, heartburn, faintness, shortness of breath, nausea, fatigue, swollen legs, sore pelvis, and throbbing feet, then you had better not give me any shit.

Yesterday, while standing in line to return a broken clock (item #74 on that massive to-do list), an impatient woman tried to elbow her way past me to reach the counter first. I turned an evil eye at her and said, "Don't you fucking dare." She silently recoiled and took her place back in line.

I can't imagine having the gall to do that under normal circumstances, but I must admit that at the time, it felt damn good!

Well, the full moon has come and gone, and still nothing. No more signs of prelabor. No signs of real labor. Nada.

Now that we have discussed what things to look for at the onset of labor, you are probably wondering what real labor actually feels like (if this is your first pregnancy, of course). Unfortunately, there are no set rules on what labor feels like. It is different for every woman, and even with every pregnancy. (Aren't you getting sick of that line? It would be nice to have some solid facts once in a while.) The best I can do is to tell you what it was like for me and some of my friends.

I remember thinking that the contractions felt like hard period/back pains, but for short periods of time (about a minute). During the contraction, I was physically unable to do any more than concentrate on my breathing.

While walking into the hospital, I had to stop every fifteen feet or so to have a contraction and breathe. The contractions were so intense that I wasn't able to answer any of the doctor's questions until the contraction was over.

Clara said her contractions during labor were more like a stabbing, concentrated back pain. Her baby's head was tilted back toward the spine, putting pressure on it every time she had a contraction. This is known as "back labor."

Jane said she felt the pain of contractions all throughout her midsection, plus it radiated down her legs and arms. She was so upset about how much pain she was having that she panicked, which only made matters worse. The more pain she felt, the more convinced she became that something was wrong. The more panicked she became, the more intense and painful her contractions became as well. She was caught in a vicious cycle. Jane's doctor suggested that it might be in the best interests of everyone to have a cesarean section as soon as possible. Jane promptly agreed and had a healthy baby girl shortly thereafter.

My friend Marsha, on the other hand, had the most casual labor of anyone I know. She was having what she thought were

Braxton Hicks contractions for a few hours. She thought it would be fun to start timing them, as if it were real labor, to practice for the big event. She soon noticed a steady pattern forming—contractions lasting about a minute, every six minutes apart, every five minutes, every four minutes, every three minutes. Hmmmm. This seemed strange. She called her doctor and told him what had been happening. Her doctor told her to get to the hospital so she could get checked out just in case.

Marsha casually walked to the hospital, all the while having her mild contractions. Upon arrival, she found the waiting area filled with several pregnant women in hard labor. When she was called in for her turn, there were many protests and shouts from the snarling mouths of labor-ridden women. They didn't think it was fair that she see a doctor first. "She couldn't possibly be in labor! Just look at that grin on her face!"

By the time Marsha saw her doctor, she was fully dilated and ready to push. Pop! Out came the baby.

I wish it could be that easy for all of us!

38

Week Forty, Patience Is a Virtue . . . and All That Crap

Symptoms: Braxton Hicks contractions, heartburn, faintness, shortness of breath, nausea, fatigue, swollen legs, sore pelvis, throbbing feet, stabbing back pain

The new symptom of the week is another variation of stabbing back pain. The left side of my lower back is continually sore and sporadically spasms, sending knifelike pains through my spine and down my leg. It is so sudden and shocking that I often drop whatever I'm carrying, or almost fall to my knees. This is certainly no time to be going out in public. I have envisioned nightmarish scenarios of strangers rushing to my aid as I have a spasm while crossing the street and forcibly admitting me to the hospital.

My friend Bridget had so many episodes of strong Braxton Hicks contractions toward the end of her pregnancy that a stranger mistook them for real labor and tried to drag her into his car to get to the hospital. When her contraction was over, she batted the man over the head with her purse and spat, "Mind your own business, buster!"

I am now officially overdue by a few days. I never thought that the second baby might be late too. I was convinced that this one

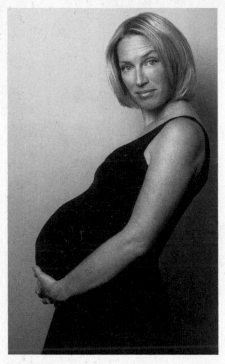

would be early to make up for how late I was with Karmen—ten freakin' days! I pray I do not have to endure that again!

Most first-time mothers fantasize that their baby will be born on the exact due date and make all plans accordingly. In reality, that rarely happens—some babies are born before, some after.

When you mark your calendar and see that date come and go, it can be quite discouraging. It almost feels as if you are being stood up by a blind date. It feels like life is put on hold. You don't want to make any plans, just in case your date decides to show. The more time that passes, the more dejected and discouraged you become. I guess the best advice is to just carry on with life as usual. Your date will show eventually, whether you are ready or not.

I'm not suggesting booking a trip to the Bahamas or anything, but try to keep yourself busy with smaller tasks and pleasures—get a pedicure, get your hair done, pay the bills, have lunch with your girlfriends, read a book, prepare thank-you notes for the baby gifts to come.

It seems that nothing is ever definite about pregnancy and childbirth. I was surprised when a nurse told me that is not the case. She said, "One thing will definitely happen to a pregnant woman—a baby will come out. One way or another, one day or another."

Yeah, yeah, it's true . . . and patience is a virtue . . . and all that crap.

While we are twiddling our thumbs, are you sure you really are ready to go? Do you have a game plan for getting to the hospital? Who's going to bring you? Whom do you need to call?

Is your hospital bag packed? Of course some things will be left to the last minute, but you can get semiready for your date.

Here is my list of what to bring to the hospital:

Insurance info. Bring your insurance card and/or telephone contact information. Most insurance companies require you to contact them within twenty-four hours of the birth, or medical expenses for the baby will not be covered.

It seems so unfair, doesn't it?

After having a long and difficult birth, Nicole had trouble reaching her insurance company within the allotted twenty-four hours. The line was continually busy. After numerous hours she finally got a live person on the phone. She ended the call with, "Yes, me, my baby, and my big, bloody vagina are doing just fine, thank you very much!"

Cord blood collection kit. This is a fairly new procedure that we have opted for, mainly because there is a high rate of cancer in our family. The baby's umbilical cord blood (with the purest form of stem cells) will be collected and then sent to a storage facility for possible further use in treating cancers or illnesses of the baby or a family member.

To find out more about cord blood, see the following Web sites:

Alpha Cord
www.alphacord.com

California CRYOBANK
www.mycordblood.com

CBR Cord Blood Registry (my choice)
www.cordblood.com

CordPartners
www.cordpartners.com

Lifebank USA—Cord Blood
www.lifebankUSA.com

Securacell
www.securacell.com

Viacord
www.viacord.com

Camera, cassette tape recorder, tapes. I intend to document all stages of the experience through labor and delivery. Unfortunately, most hospitals, mine included, don't allow videotaping. My digital camera does take small video clips, but you would never be able to tell just by looking at it. It's quite small and looks like a regular instamatic camera. Shhhhh. Don't tell.

Lollipops. Although you are generally not allowed to have anything to eat during labor and delivery, sometimes hard candies are permitted to keep your mouth moist and give you a small sugar boost. I have found lollipops to be more permissible than regular hard candies because there is less risk of choking on something with a stick attached to it.

Snacks for the coach. You will be unable to partake, but your partner/labor coach will need some nourishment eventually. Who knows how long labor will last? It could be just a few minutes, several hours, or even days. The last thing you want is your coach to be leaving you for a "quick bite to eat" when you are in the final stages of ghastly labor.

Unless you have a minicooler for cold drinks and nonperishable foods, it's usually best to bring items that don't require refrigeration, as you never know if you are going to be able to store your snack in the hospital fridge. You also might want to pack some extra change for the hospital vending machines.

Also, Grace insists that I remind you, definitely no breath-smelly foods allowed for the coach. Her husband David's Dorito breath significantly contributed to her nausea and contempt for him during labor.

Socks. Your feet will probably get cold because the delivery room is usually kept fairly cool. Be sure to bring a few pairs of socks, as blood and other fluids may soak them from time to time. This may seem alarming, but believe me, this is yet another one of those things that you will look back on as no big deal.

Slippers. If your feet are not looking up to snuff, I suggest the closed-toe slipper. We don't want to subject our visitors to our long, yellowing toenails on blistered, wart- or corn-riddled feet, do we?

Panties. Pack as many as you can. You may go through a lot if you have an extended stay. Also, I find it very important to pack at least two pairs of maternity underwear. Even if you haven't given in to wearing them throughout your entire pregnancy, you still may need them in the event you have a C-section.

My friend Camilla was dead set against maternity underwear. She was convinced her husband would never have sex with her again if he saw her wearing those bloomers. When she found herself in the hospital after a C-section with no maternity underwear, she called me in desperation. Her regular underwear was cutting into her abdomen, right where the incision was, and she had to wear panties to keep a sanitary pad in place. "Bring me some freakin' bloomers, please!"

PJs. It is nice to have your own PJs, but I do not recommend putting them on until after the birth—they may get a bit messy.

Some women prefer to wear the hospital gowns during their whole stay, but I find them to be cumbersome while trying to navigate the bathroom with a room full of guests. The back never stays closed enough to cover your tush, especially when you still have a swollen middle.

If you plan on breast-feeding, bring PJs that button down the front for easy booby access. I made that mistake the first time around and had to awkwardly navigate my nipple through the neck or armhole for feedings.

Comfortable bras for sleeping. If you are in the hospital long enough to have your milk come in (usually forty-eight hours after the birth), it is important to have some kind of support for your breasts. When the milk comes in, watch out, breasts can get humongous.

If you have ever contemplated getting breast implants, here is your chance to see what the XXL size would look like. Your breasts will swell to the maximum capacity of the skin and become as hard as rocks. Not only is this painful, but it is a lot harder to get the baby to "latch on" to a rock than a soft nipple. Wearing a snug yet comfortable bra at least limits some of the expansion of the milk ducts.

Pillows. As I mentioned earlier, hospital pillows are usually pretty flimsy and scratchy. It's also nice to have some comforts of home in your hospital bed. Make sure you bring colored or patterned pillowcases so that your pillows do not get mixed up with the hospital's white laundry.

If you have any teenagers around, make sure they don't mess with your pillows. Nicole's nephew inserted a whoopee cushion into her pillowcase. He was quite satisfied when he found out that the nurse, Jessie, endured much humiliation from his prank. The room full of guests assumed she was the one tooting while helping adjust Nicole's pillows.

Toiletries. You know, your regular traveling stuff: toothpaste, deodorant, lotions, makeup, and so on.

Phone list. It's a good idea to prioritize your list of people to call, with their phone numbers, into a few categories.

- People to call when you go into labor. These people may want to be at the hospital for the actual birth—close friends and/or family members in front of whom you don't mind losing your composure. I clearly remember Nicole screaming, "You bloody, fucking baaaaaastaaaaaards!!!" while her mother and I clenched white-knuckled hands in the hallway.

    Do remember that your coach and/or partner should be on top of this phone list. When Hannah went into labor, she was so busy with her "list of people to call" that she forgot to notify her husband. Her contractions suddenly were five minutes apart, he hadn't been notified, and he was more than thirty minutes away. The garbage-man brought her to the hospital.

- People to call after the baby is born. These are close friends and/or family you want to share the news with immediately, the people who want to be kept abreast of the situation, no matter what time of the day—or night—it is. My sister was delighted to be awoken at 4:30 A.M. for the news of Karmen's birth.

- People to call after the baby is born (at a reasonable hour).

- People to call during your hospital stay. Calls that you can make if and when you feel like it.

Calling card and/or change for phone. Most hospital pay phones and in-room phones don't allow long-distance calls. It's wise to be prepared with plenty of change and/or a calling card.

Be aware that cell phones in the hospital are usually not an option. If you are caught using a cell phone, expect the full wrath of the nurses to come down on you. Believe me, this is no time to be pissing off the nurses!

Going-home outfit for you and baby. My friend Ava envisioned her and her baby returning home in their matching Laura Ashley mother-daughter outfits. Her dress was so tight that she caught a good hunk of back fat in the zipper that required the nurse's assistance to remove. And the scratchy, linen material of the baby's dress made her newborn skin break out in hives.

Of course you and your baby want to look your best for your first appearance into the outside world together, but, as with pregnancy, comfort should be key.

Keep in mind that you will not automatically fit into your pre-maternity clothes. It may take several weeks for your bowl-of-jelly belly to return to its former shape. It might be best to bring some of your more flattering, not-so-maternity-looking maternity clothes. You know, not the circus tent, just the pup tent should suffice.

39

Week Forty-Plus, Five Freakin' Days and Counting . . .

At my weekly doctor's appointment, I learned that I am now two centimeters dilated. I guess the Braxton Hicks contractions are accomplishing something. While I was being examined, my doctor told me he was going to strip my membranes. Ewww. What does that mean? It sounded painful.

It was a little uncomfortable, as all pelvic exams are at this point, but not painful. My doctor ran his fingers all around the inner edges of the cervix to disengage any attached membranes to maybe, we hoped, facilitate labor.

He also told me that, since I am now five (freakin') days overdue, if I did not deliver by Monday, I should come in for a fetal stress test and a sonogram. These tests determine if the baby is maintaining a good heart rate and has enough amniotic fluid surrounding her. Depending on the test results, I will be able to wait a few days more, have a C-section scheduled, or have my water broken to induce labor.

Because I am going for the VBAC, inducing labor is not usually recommended, but since I am already dilating, the breaking of membranes is okay, I guess. No Pitocin allowed, though. (I am

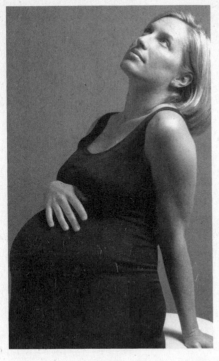

grateful for this, as I remember the drug making labor pains much more intense and erratic with the last pregnancy.)

Last night at about 9 P.M., contractions began. They were lasting about one minute and were ten minutes apart for a few hours. This could be "it," or at least maybe the precursor to "it."

The only reason I wasn't completely convinced that it was real labor was the fact that the contractions were not as strong (painful) as I remembered. I was able to talk and move during the contractions. Maybe they would get stronger when they became closer together, or maybe I would get lucky and experience just a mildly uncomfortable labor and delivery, like Marsha. Ha! I won't hold my breath, though.

I went to bed at 11 P.M. and was able to doze, on and off, until about 1:30 A.M., which is when the contractions became too intense to ignore. I had to practice the Lamaze breathing to get through them, and they were now every six minutes apart . . . then every five minutes apart . . . then every four.

My doctor told me to call if my contractions were less than ten minutes apart, but was this the real thing? I didn't want to be sent home after checking into the hospital. (If this is your first delivery and you are experiencing steady contractions (mild or not) of five minutes apart or less, call your doctor. You never know if your labor is going to be a Jane or a Marsha version. If Marsha didn't call the doctor when she did, she might have delivered on a New York City sidewalk.)

I was trying to be quiet, but I guess my huffy, Lamaze breathing woke Jamey again. "Is it time to go to the hospital?" he asked.

"No, no. I'm pretty sure it's false labor."

He rolled over and went back to sleep.

During my first pregnancy, we were both awake through the first forty-eight hours of what we thought was real labor. Jamey had the stopwatch to time the contractions and stood by to make sure I was doing the Lamaze breathing properly. At 3 A.M., the contractions were less than three minutes apart. We notified the first "tier" on the phone list, packed it up, and got to the hospital.

I was checked in, but by morning my contractions had slowed from two minutes to five minutes apart. I was diagnosed with false labor and only two centimeters dilated, so they told me to go home. I should not come back until my water broke, or the contractions were less than one minute apart.

Go home!? I was ready to have this baby today!

The contractions didn't completely stop, but they turned into real labor within a few days.

If I am following the same pattern, this potentially false labor may be the precursor of my real labor.

Well, I was right. It was false labor. By 4 A.M., the contractions had ceased and I was finally able to get some sleep.

So here I am today, no more contractions and . . . still waiting.

Last night was the same story: false labor that kept me awake for a few hours and then ceased.

This morning I have one more sign of labor to report. Ta-dah! I have lost the mucous plug. It must mean that my cervix is dilating farther and things are progressing.

Still, no real labor to report.

Jamey suggested that we go for a brisk walk this morning to stir things up.

It would be nice to have the labor and delivery during the day,

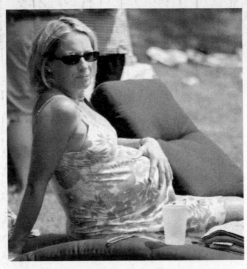

"Has anyone got some Tums?"

instead of having to wake up ol' grouchy bear to drive me to the hospital. I think Jamey would be particularly annoyed if his precious slumber was disturbed by yet another round of false labor.

Well, the walk didn't help and we are still waiting.

Again, more false labor. I certainly am getting tired of this!

This morning I had some "bloody show" and quite a bit of thick mucous discharge. All normal, all signs of pending labor. But when are we going to get on with the "show"? When?

40

Week Forty-one, Doing
It My Way

Finally, last night, after many hours of false labor contractions, I settled into bed. That's when the real contractions started. I was suddenly startled by a large kick from the baby, immediately followed by a real contraction. Yes! A real contraction! Welcome to me!

How did I know it was a real contraction? Well, it spread from my lower back and encompassed my whole middle. My uterus then became extremely tight, distorted looking, and painful. I noticed at the height of the contraction that I had a few waves of nausea from the pain. I can see why some women vomit during labor. Again, the Lamaze breathing really helped me distance the pain and get through it.

Jamey kept asking me, "Is this real labor? Is this it? Is it? Is it? Is it?!" The clincher for me was the fact that I could not talk during a contraction. This was definitely it! We started timing the contractions and soon noticed that they were progressing very quickly. By 11:30 they were already six minutes apart. Uh-oh . . . we should have already been at the hospital.

I packed my last-minute items and grabbed a bunch of old towels for the car (you never know when your water may break).

By the time the babysitter arrived, the contractions were five minutes apart.

I, for one, was happy to have things progressing so quickly. Jamey, on the other hand, was looking a bit ashen. We arrived at the hospital by midnight. As we approached the nurses' desk, I blurted out, "Epidural," before Jamey could even begin to tell her my name. I wanted to be clear that this was a top priority.

It seemed Jamey's top priority was to get me admitted, and fast. Although I was already preadmitted, there still were a few forms to fill out. The panic on Jamey's face finally diminished when I was hooked up to all the proper monitors and was fully in the care of the hospital staff.

By the time the doctor examined me, at 1:30 A.M., I was already six centimeters dilated. Yeah! Epidural time! (Most hospitals have a standard of at least four to five centimeters' dilation required before it can be administered.)

Upon voicing my request of the epidural to my doctor, he advised me against it. He told me that in his opinion, with a VBAC delivery, an epidural could diminish the chances of a vaginal birth by about 30 percent. The drug sometimes interferes with a mother's ability to push.

What?! I was never told this before. I had come into this hospital with a plan and thought that I had already made all my decisions. What should we do now? At that moment, another contraction seized my uterus. Presto! My mind was made up. It was epidural time. No matter how numb the epidural made me feel, I would *find* a way to push.

Once my decision was made, I still had to get through over an hour more of contractions. Before an epidural can be administered, you have to get a bag of IV juice pumped into you, someone has to summon the anesthesiologist, the anesthesiologist has to brief you on the procedure, and then, finally, you get to have the big needle in the spine. By the time I was ready for my spinal poke, at about 3 A.M., I was already seven centimeters dilated and starting the "transition" stage of labor. At that point,

the contractions became more intense and my body was beginning to shake.

This time, when the anesthesiologist swabbed my back with
antiseptic, I was actually looking forward to having that needle
jabbed into my spine. The first injection of novocaine was a small
pinch that was no more uncomfortable than having blood drawn.
The second injection, where the anesthesiologist puts a larger
needle into the spinal column and inserts a tiny catheter, didn't
hurt at all. It just felt kind of strange, as if someone was poking
around inside my back.

Believe it or not, the most painful part of the epidural was afterward, when the ductlike tape was torn off my back.

Suddenly, my right leg gave a wild kick as I felt a jolt, a cold
and electric feeling but not painful, go from my hip to my toes.
And . . . that was it. No more pain. "Am I having a contraction?"
I asked as I felt a pressure and squeezing of my uterus.

"A huge one," Jamey replied as he turned the monitor my way
so that I could see the blue line spike off the chart.

At 5:15 A.M. the doctor examined me and announced that I
was fully dilated and ready to push. Great! Let's get this show on
the road! Jamey stepped into the bathroom for a quick break, the
doctor left the room to get his scrubs, and the nurse disappeared
down the hall. I felt my next contraction taking hold and I was all
alone. Should I start pushing? Hello? I was about to have a baby
here! By the time the contraction was at its height, the room was
full of people again and I was back in the spotlight.

The nurse coached me on my pushing and assigned Jamey a
few tasks—supporting my neck and right leg during contractions, and giving me the oxygen mask after each push. The nurse
kept telling me to push out through my rectum, as if having a giant bowel movement. I guess that is the closest feeling you can
compare it to. During one very hard push, I heard a fart escape.
Egads! "Did I poop?" I asked in horror. No, the nurse assured me,
it was just a sign that I was doing it right. It wasn't a fart; it was
what she called "baby bubbles."

During that mildly embarrassing episode, I was grateful that it was just the nurse and Jamey in the room. Believe it or not, in most hospitals the doctor is not present much of the time during the labor and even the pushing stages. That was fine with me. I found the nurses to be fully capable and encouraging throughout the entire birthing process.

After a few hard pushes, the nurse announced that she could see the baby's head. Of course, I couldn't see from my angle, but I could feel the baby's head beginning to peek out. Jamey became so mesmerized that he forgot to give me oxygen.

"Jamey, oxygen," the nurse said.

Although the baby's head was becoming more visible with each push, it kept sucking back in every time I stopped. It felt as if I was severely constipated. Maybe I should hold the push until the next contraction? Was that possible?

The doctor made occasional visits to see how I was progressing and each time expressed dissatisfaction with my progress. The baby's head was not advancing down the birth canal fast enough.

During my next push, the doctor asked the nurse for a long, pointy instrument. "What is that? What the hell are you doing?" I wanted to say, but I had no air to speak. He reached in and I suddenly felt a warm wetness. Oh, it was just the water bag he broke.

"Jamey, oxygen," the nurse reminded.

The doctor said if I didn't deliver within two hours, he recommended the C-section, as an extended strain on the uterus could put too much stress on the former scar. I looked at the clock. Where did the time go!? I had only forty-five minutes to get the baby out. This doctor was really beginning to irritate me.

After the doctor left the room, the nurse warned me that the epidural was about to wear off. The medication being fed into the catheter was almost gone and she was sure the doctor would not allow me another dose. I heard a windy, swooshing noise in my head. Sounds in the room were becoming distant. The one thing I did hear, loud and clear, was Jamey's voice, "Push!" And I did, as

hard as I could. The baby's head was advancing, but soooooo
slowly.

"Jamey, oxygen."

Just after the two-hour limit, the doctor returned. His mouth
flattened into one thin line and he shook his head from side to
side. On my next contraction, I summoned up all the energy I
could muster and pushed like hell.

"DON'T YOU DARE SHAKE YOUR CONTEMPTUOUS HEAD
AT MEEEEEEEEEEEEEEEE!!!"

I was really starting to feel those contraction pains again, but
the baby was progressing.

"Jamey, oxygen."

After I got my breath back, I asked, "Please give me more
time," in my most reasonable voice. If I could convince him that
I was a cooperative patient and he was the one in control, maybe
I could continue to do things my way.

Since the baby's heart rate was stable and I was still going
strong with the pushing, I was given an extra thirty minutes. After that, if the baby was not born, I would be scheduled for the
first surgery of the day, at 7:30 A.M.

The hands on the clock advanced quickly. The doctor would
be back any minute, the epidural was done, and the baby was still
not out. Oh shit. Oh shit. Oh shit!

The nurse positioned a mirror so that I could see my progress
with each push. I saw the top of the baby's head, with lots of
black hair, trying to burst free. If I could just get her out . . . I
somehow managed to push a little harder and the baby moved a
little more.

"Jamey, oxygen."

Oh, no. The doctor was back. He moved the mirror out of the
way, checked on my progress, and announced it was time for the
surgery. "NO WAY! I can do it!" I screamed, now unable to sup-
press my raging will. I mean, "Just give me a little more time," I
pleaded in my most respectful voice.

Jamey then interjected a bit of buddy-boy golf banter, which helped soften the mood. At the time, I was wondering, What the hell does golf have to do with the price of tomatoes? We managed to convince the doctor to schedule us for the second surgery of the day.

I continued to push, harder and harder, and the baby kept progressing. With each push I was becoming more and more out of breath. I barely had enough energy to slap Jamey in the chest.

"Jamey, oxygen."

When the doctor returned, I was finally close to delivery. Before the next contraction took hold, I asked if it was possible to avoid an episiotomy. The thought of having to be cut from my vagina to rectum was giving me the heebie-jeebies.

The doctor suppressed a laugh and said that waiting for the stretching of the perineum could add hours to the delivery. I guess that meant avoiding the episiotomy was not an option.

So I'm sprawled out on my back, spread-eagle, with my swollen vagina hanging out, and he's being smug with me? Maybe he's pissed because it looks like he won't get to do the C-section after all. Okay. Fine. I'll let him do one small operation to satisfy his scalpelitis.

> **Dr. Miriam Greene says:** It's my experience that most OB/GYNs are compassionate and caring throughout the birthing process and don't have "scalpelitis." Do choose your doctor carefully. Trust your gut.

It actually was not bad at all. I was surprised that with the epidural worn off, I didn't even feel the injection of novocaine before the cut was made.

With the next contraction, I gave another hard push and suddenly felt some relief of pressure. The nurses and doctor huddled in closer, and Jamey leaned over to get a better look too. What is going on down there? I wondered, as I let my breath out and tried to lift my head.

"The head is out!" Jamey announced. I tried to peek around the still-large orb of my belly, but my vision was obstructed by the hands of the doctor. "Keep pushing," he said, as he grabbed the baby's head and turned her body.

I took another deep breath, held it, and gave another hard push. This time I felt no resistance, and the baby's small body slid out in one smooth motion.

She is out. I did it! I somehow found the strength to get her out and into this world. The doctor held the baby up.

And you thought I wouldn't be able to have a vaginal birth! Told you so! I would have spit in his face if I weren't so damn happy.

I heard the cries of the baby and saw the nurse suction some goop out of her mouth. Within seconds, she was placed on my stomach.

She was small and slimy, with a slightly gray tone to her skin, but she was so beautiful. This glowing life force was crying, flailing her floppy arms and legs around, and looking at me. She was so small, so helpless. "What is going on here?" her eyes seemed to be asking me.

I reached down and held her tiny body, gook and all. Her flailing calmed to some mild twitches and she turned her glossy, round face up to me. I stroked my fingers across her grapefruit-sized head, covered with a good amount of thick, dark hair, and noticed that she didn't have a cone head.

I have seen many vaginally delivered babies with a cone-head appearance that sometimes lasts days after the birth. The plates of bone in the baby's skull usually shift to allow the passage through the birth canal. Strange that her skull bones didn't shift. Maybe that's why it was so hard to get the head out.

I traced my fingertips down the side of her face, and her quivering lower lip, on her tiny M-shaped mouth became still. She has my mouth. This little person was my baby. She reached her

tiny hand toward mine and
grabbed hold of my little
finger. What long, delicate
fingers she had. I wonder
what side of the family
those are from.

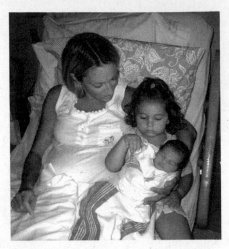

The light in the room
must have been quite a
shock to her newborn eyes.
She repeatedly tried to open
them wide and had to
squint against the glare.
The irises of her eyes were
already a very dark brown,
like pools of balsamic vine-

Isn't it worth it? Devon Sloan, born 8:15 A.M.,
8 pounds, 20 inches

gar on china-white plates. At that moment, she was so beautiful
to me that I felt like I could devour her. Maybe that is why cats
constantly lick their newborn kittens.

This time, the love I felt for the baby was instant. With Karmen's birth it took me a few days to be coherent enough even to
get a good look at her. What a difference between a vaginal and a
C-birth!

The nurse then whisked the baby away for a quick cleanup.

Then the doctor stitched up my perineum. Thank goodness
for novocaine!

Next came the delivery of the afterbirth. With a minimal
amount of pushing, the placenta came sliding out. The doctor
held it up for me to get a good look at it. I began to laugh, as I
thought it looked like my liver had just fallen out, except that it
had a phone cord attached to it. The nurse gave me a strange look
as she handed me my baby. I guess she didn't see the humor in a
placenta.

Jamey stood close and put his hands on the baby, too, as I drew
her in for her first breast-feeding. Although I had experienced it

before, I was amazed that she seemed to know just what to do—
as if she had been suckling many times before.

I envisioned a scene from Dr. Seuss's *The Grinch Who Stole
Christmas*. The Grinch's tiny heart grew and grew until it burst
out of its tight wire frame. And he felt, for the very first time, real
love.

41

Nineteen Days After, Hypothesis False

So here I am, three weeks after the baby was born and still in the throes of baby slavery. Don't get me wrong—it's not all bad. There is the almost sickening joy of the growing love for my baby. It seems as if it oozes from her each time I cuddle her curved little body under my chin, infecting me with the baby-love virus. It is truly a wonderful disease!

The euphoria of this love plague does help balance out the fatigue, but it is still trying at times. Finding time for myself has been a real challenge. The good news is I am seeing signs of things getting easier. Devon is starting to form sleeping and eating patterns, which enables me to schedule my time more efficiently. After her late morning feeding, she usually sleeps for an hour or more, which is my window of opportunity to take a shower, get some work done, or write another chapter.

While reflecting back on my daughter's birth, I have to say I am quite satisfied that I was able to do the VBAC. I had the experience of childbirth both ways—a VBAC victory! When the doctor was once again urging me to get the C-section, I was also thinking of you, my friend. I thought a book like this would be better served if I could give a personal account of a cesarean and a vaginal birth. I considered, just for a moment, telling him that another C would be anticlimactic for my book. Did he really want to be the cause of my publishing downfall?

When I recall my experience of pain and feelings of anxiety during labor and delivery, I can honestly say that my memories are now very vague and foggy. I do remember having pain, but I don't quite remember what it felt like. When I try to recall the sensation, it's as if my brain is searching for some distant file that is close to being fully deleted, like a fading dream on the morning after. Upon rereading the details of Devon's birth, my memory is momentarily restored, but it soon fades again. It seems as if some-one is definitely trying to erase that file. So I was wrong—it is true that time does fade the memories of childbirth pain (at least in my case). I am so glad that I was able to get down the details of the birth before they faded away.

Here's some good news about the pain of a vaginal childbirth. I originally thought that the vaginal area would be the most painful during the delivery and found that not to be the case at all. Most women agree that the vaginal area during childbirth be-comes naturally numb from the continual pressure of the baby bearing down.

If you haven't had your baby yet, you are probably wondering what your actual childbirth experience will be like. Will it be like mine? Will you have a vaginal birth or a C-section? Will you have an easy Marsha labor, or will it be a prolonged Jane version? What will the pains of labor be like for you?

If it's any consolation, even during the most difficult parts of my labors and deliveries, I knew that I would gladly go through it all again to have another child. The rewards greatly outweigh the seemingly minor discomforts of pregnancy and childbirth.

And when you have someone to go through it with you every step of the way, it can actually be fun: to laugh at each other's un-controllable flatulence, to compare the size of hemorrhoids, to confess tirades of hormone-driven behavior, and to share in the scary yet exciting experience of childbirth and motherhood.

It's always more fun to go on a roller-coaster ride with a good friend. Don't you agree?

THE END.

But really just the beginning . . .

Part Two

· · · · · · · · · · · · ·

REAL QUESTIONS, REAL ANSWERS

Here's a collection of questions and answers selected from my Web site, FranklyPregnant.com. This is not a compilation of comprehensive or frequently asked questions. These are not the Q&As you will find in just about every other pregnancy book. These are the embarrassing questions. The odd and unusual questions. The questions people don't like to ask, let alone discuss. Some of it is gross, some of it is shocking, but most of it is pretty funny. Enjoy!

Although Dr. Greene does add her commentary and suggestions throughout these Q&As, you should consult with your own doctor about any unusual symptoms or pregnancy concerns, especially if they involve bleeding, pain, fainting or dizziness, fever, excess vomiting, or diarrhea.

42

Belly Issues

Q. I was sitting on a chair at work and bent forward to pick up a pen off the floor. As I did, I felt a crunching (like that of two bones being rubbed together) in my tummy where the baby's head is. Is it possible that I may have caused damage?

A. This crunching, rubbing, bag-of-rocks-in-the-belly feeling is normal. Before I was ever "with child" I remember thinking that a pregnant belly would be very much like having a fat stomach. I found quite the contrary to be true. Unlike soft, pliable fat, my stomach felt like it was filled with a bag of rocks that crunched against my ribs and pelvic bones when I bent over or squatted. Don't worry; the baby is well protected and quite pliable. After all, the baby's head and body will get squished considerably more during childbirth.

Q. Sometimes my husband will try to feel the baby move, and if he can't feel anything, he will jiggle my belly and she will kick. Will this cause any damage? I feel silly asking my doctor, and don't want to offend my husband and tell him to stop.

A. I don't think you need be concerned. The baby is well cushioned within your uterus and surrounded by amniotic fluid. A vigorous shaking of the belly is probably no more jarring than a gentle nudge.

I, too, remember shaking the belly to wake my baby so that my friends and family could feel her move. I think it's a pretty common practice among expecting parents.

> **Dr. Miriam Greene says:** I sometimes use an acoustic stimulator to wake a sleeping baby, as well as a little shake.

Q. Is it harmful to the baby if I sleep on my belly? I am fifteen weeks pregnant.

A. I don't think you need to worry. The baby is surrounded by plenty of amniotic fluid and padding and won't be able to tell the difference between sleeping on your back, side, or belly.

I recommend sleeping on your belly as much as possible while you still can. In a few weeks it will be very uncomfortable, and in a few months it will be physically impossible. As the months go by, you will find that sleeping on your left side is the most comfortable position and promotes optimum circulation, which is beneficial to you and your baby. During my last pregnancy, I longed to be able to lie on my belly. I remedied the situation with a trip to the beach every now and then. I dug a big pit in the sand, threw my towel over it, and then was able to finally rest, sunny-side down.

Q. My baby is amazingly active throughout the night. As soon as I lie down, the baby thinks it's time to party. I can't sleep through this baby mambo. Is there anything I can do?

A. In-utero babies are usually the most active a few hours after the mother has eaten. That's when the baby gets his or her infusion of nutrients and sugars via the umbilical cord. Perhaps you should have your dinner earlier so that the baby may do so as well. Having your largest meal of the day at midday could also prove to be helpful.

During the day, a mother's voice and movements can be quite soothing, allowing the baby to sleep more. Short of sleeping in a moving vehicle, you could try a vibrating mattress or mattress pad.

I hate to tell you this, but if you're having trouble sleeping now, you're really going to be sleepless in a few months when backache, heartburn, constant peeing, leg cramps, and nightmares set in.

Q. I have a bruise on my pelvic area. Could it be from the baby kicking?

A. If you see a bruise on your skin, it's probably not the baby's kicks that caused it. If the baby bruised anything at all, it would be the uterine lining, which you wouldn't see but might feel.

> **Dr. Miriam Greene says:** Lots of veins come to the surface of the abdomen during pregnancy and are very prone to rupturing, which can cause a bruise.

It's quite common during pregnancy to become very klutzy, especially while carrying around a big ol' belly that you're not used to navigating. It's possible that you hit your hip or pelvis on a table or something without even realizing it. It happens *a lot* during pregnancy.

Q. The right side of my lower abdomen has been very tender to the touch. I can also feel something hard behind it when I touch it. What is this? Do I need to be worried?

A. What you are experiencing is normal, and yes, I've had it too. I called it "the sore spot syndrome." These tender spots on the uterus are usually localized to one area and remain for a few days at a time before moving on to another spot. When I had a Braxton Hicks contraction, the sore spot was the most painful. Sometimes the baby puts a lot of pressure on a certain area of the uterus, making it tender and sensitive, like a bruise, or the baby can push on certain nerve endings, which has the same effect. The hardness you felt is probably the baby's back, head, or behind pushing on that tender area.

Q. I'm thirty-nine weeks pregnant and have a sharp pain under my ribs. What could this be?

A. I would guess that the baby is kicking you in the ribs. In the last few weeks, space is usually limited and the baby is becoming stronger and more active. I can remember, on quite a few occasions, having to reach in under my rib to dislodge my baby's foot, which was painfully pressing on my diaphragm. The good news is, if you are feeling feet in your ribs, then the baby is head down, not a breech position, and ready to go.

Q. I am eight months pregnant and sometimes my stomach feels as hard as a rock. There are other times when I can feel the different parts of the baby and some soft, fluidy areas. Is this normal?

A. When your uterus is relaxed, you might be able to decipher where your baby's head, back, or feet are within the soft surroundings. At the times when your stomach is feeling rock-hard, you are probably having a Braxton Hicks contraction. Sometimes you may feel cramping or pressure during a Braxton Hicks and sometimes you won't. These contractions can last anywhere from a few seconds to several minutes.

Q. I'm getting married soon and have just discovered I'm pregnant! I already have my dress, which requires a corset. Is it safe to wear a steel-boned corset, laced loosely, at week thirteen of a pregnancy?

A. As long as the corset doesn't make you uncomfortable, deprive you of oxygen, or make you feel overheated, I think you will be fine. You need to trust your gut on this one—if it doesn't feel right, don't wear it. Unfortunately, you probably won't be able to tell for sure until your big day. If the dress doesn't work without the corset, you may want to have an alternate outfit just in case.

43

Body Odors

Q. I've been experiencing an odor coming from between my breasts, and even my husband notices the smell. I've resorted to putting deodorant between my boobs. I take two showers a day, but immediately after I bathe the odor is there again. What do you think is causing this? How can I make it go away? It's so embarrassing!

A. During pregnancy, most women not only have different body odor, but they also smell stronger. It's the horror-mones of pregnancy that change your body's chemistry and scent. You may also notice that you perspire from places you never have before—like between your breasts. I remember having sweaty shins during my first pregnancy. It was really embarrassing when I had a pedicure and the sweat kept rolling down onto my feet.

Back to the issue of odors and how to control them: The good news is that once the baby is born, you will probably get your old scent back. The bad news is that you may have to tolerate your different odor until your pregnancy is over.

To lessen the scent, you might try a slightly blander diet with minimal garlic or spicy foods that can be a catalyst for stinky

sweat. You also might try using a corn-starch-based powder between your boobs. Powder formulated for foot odor may work
best, as it absorbs moisture and deodorizes.

Q. My wife says she can't stand the smell of me, although I
shower three times a day and wear deodorants. She won't even
sleep in the same bedroom. Any suggestions?

A. The horror-mones of pregnancy can wreak havoc on a woman's
olfactory sensors, turning the volume way up on smells. Some
women have more of a "smelling" problem than others. My
friend Hannah slept in a separate bedroom throughout her entire
pregnancy. She said the smell of her husband's sleep/morning
breath was so offensive that she would vomit upon whiffing it.
You are not alone.

Try not to feel offended. Sometimes during pregnancy any
smell in close contact can be repugnant. It's a good idea to bathe
often to keep your scent to a minimum. Since just the showering
isn't doing the trick, maybe you should investigate just what it is
that is not agreeing with your wife's nose. Maybe it's your deodorant or cologne. Maybe it's the smell of a spicy or garlic-filled food
that you've eaten. I remember having a real problem working in
the same office as my boss the day after he ate garlic (which was
quite often). I had to light candles, open windows, and ask him
not to come within ten feet of me. That smell literally made me
sick to my stomach.

Q. Both my dog and my cat seem to want to sniff at my breasts.
I can't smell anything unusual myself, and my breasts aren't
leaking. Do you think they can smell that I'm pregnant?

A. Most animals, such as cats and dogs, have a much keener sense
of smell than we humans do. During pregnancy, I counted this as
a blessing, as I found my sense of smell to be so magnified that a

burning cigarette in a car a half mile down the road would make me ill. It's very possible that your pets are smelling changes in you, including your breasts beginning to make colostrum. Your cat and dog are probably just curious and I'm sure it's harmless sniffing. They just want to know if you're preparing to give birth or if you're stashing a quart of milk in your bra.

44

Diet and Exercise

Q. Would it be harmful to diet in the first three months? I'd like to lose about ten pounds before the second trimester comes and the weight starts to come too.

A. Unless you are obese and your doctor has told you that you must, dieting during pregnancy is not a good idea. Proper nutrition and sufficient calorie intake during the first three months are especially critical to the baby's development.

The good news is that if you're worried about becoming a big fatty, you probably won't.

I did pregnancy both ways: The first time I ate like a fiend and became quite overweight. The second time I just ate when hungry and gained twenty pounds less. Of course, the second time I was much more conscientious about what I ate, as you seem to be.

Dr. Miriam Greene says: I never recommend dieting during pregnancy.

Q. How important is it *really* to drink a lot of water when you're pregnant? I'm way too busy during the day and have not been drinking a lot. I catch up a little in the evenings and never really feel "thirsty."

A. It is recommended that you drink about two quarts of fluids a day during pregnancy. It doesn't all have to be water. Juice, decaf tea, or milk can count toward your two quarts. Is it important to follow this guideline? I think so. Your baby requires plenty of fluids to develop; your uterus, breasts, and amniotic sac become engorged with fluids; and your body is working overtime to filter out toxins (baby's waste and so on) from your system, making you urinate much more frequently. Of course, the more you drink, the more you urinate, but it's a trade-off that's well worth a healthier baby and mother.

I know it's hard to find the time in a hectic schedule to add yet one more daily task. You might try to force down two cups of water before work, then keep a bottle of water in your car, on your desk, and by your side for most of the day so when you think of it, you can take a quick sip.

P.S. When you feel "thirsty," your body is already dehydrated and that is not good for you or the baby.

Q. I am three months pregnant and want to get my butt in shape (literally). Is it safe to do lunges and squats?

A. If you haven't already been doing a particular exercise frequently, I don't think now is the time to start something new unless it's easy walking or swimming. If you've already been doing squats and lunges, you can continue as long as you are careful. Do them slowly, without quick jerky movements, and stop if you feel discomfort or out of breath. The key to monitoring your exercise level is to listen to your body. It will tell you by a contraction, dizziness, or pain when to stop.

Dr. Miriam Greene says: Only under close supervision would I advise starting a new, strenuous exercise regimen during a pregnancy.

P.S. I don't know of any woman who's been able to keep her butt in shape during pregnancy. I think it's pretty much out of your control, so don't kill yourself trying to keep your tushie tiny.

45

Harmful to the Fetus?

Q. My husband and I rented a Doppler fetal heart rate monitor. Hearing my baby's heartbeat is so reassuring. Will bouncing sound waves off my baby every day cause a problem?

A. The Doppler, a handheld ultrasound device, is not harmful to a developing fetus, as it doesn't use X-rays or other types of possibly harmful radiation. I don't think you need to worry about overusing it. Your baby probably gets more exposure to bouncing sound waves when you eat a meal or pass gas.

Q. Can I use hair bleach on my stomach?

A. To bleach or not to bleach? I faced this question during both of my pregnancies, except I was contemplating whether or not to continue my usual hair highlights. There is a common fear that bleach, hair dyes, and chemicals from permanents can be absorbed into the bloodstream, potentially harming the developing fetus.

However, studies thus far have shown that there is no link between the use of such chemicals during pregnancy and the development of birth defects. The same holds true for bleaches meant for body hair.

It's difficult to make decisions between what is pleasant for you versus what may be best for your baby. My personal feeling is that I had to give up so much in order to be a host for a life in progress, so I decided to keep my blond highlights. No harm was done.

Q. I am six weeks pregnant and have been eating spicy food throughout. Is this harmful to the baby's development?

A. If you enjoy spicy foods, go ahead and eat them while you still can. In a normal pregnancy, the baby should not be adversely affected. Later in pregnancy, you might experience the common problems of heartburn, diarrhea, gas, and bloating that can be aggravated by eating spicy foods. I remember actually having dreams about gorging on spicy Indian food during my second pregnancy. I craved it so badly but couldn't have a bite without experiencing extremely painful gas and diarrhea.

When breast-feeding, you should abstain from eating gas-causing and spicy foods. The flavors and gases from foods can be passed on through the breast milk, and newborns have extremely sensitive digestive systems.

Q. Can the stress of dealing with my four-year-old's temper tantrums be harmful to my baby or me?

A. I can certainly relate to the stress brought on by dealing with a four-year-old's tantrums. It can be especially difficult to deal with when pregnant. The horror-mones of pregnancy can make your temper's fuse extremely short and hard to control. Short-term stresses such as this can cause fatigue, sleeplessness, anxiety, poor appetite, headaches, and backaches. Only when a pregnant woman experiences very high levels of stress for an extended period could the baby be at risk for preterm labor and low birth weight.

Since I highly doubt your four-year-old is in a perpetual state of tantrums, I think you and your baby will be fine. In the meantime, you might try giving yourself time-outs during these tantrums. If your child is safe, walk out of the room, breathe, and try to relax before going back in to deal with the situation. I bet you'll be surprised at how just a few seconds of peace can make a difference in your stress level.

Q. I conceived in mid-December and attended many gatherings during the holidays in which I consumed alcohol on a regular basis. I found out I was pregnant on New Year's. I have not had any alcohol since. Will this affect my unborn baby? Some have recommended an abortion.

A. I think an abortion would be a little drastic in your case. Almost every one of my girlfriends who has borne a child had at least one (if not several) episodes of alcohol consumption during early pregnancy—mostly because they had no idea they were pregnant. It also seems that lots of people become pregnant while on vacation, which lends itself to the more-than-occasional cocktail.

If you are mentally flogging yourself for an incidental cocktail or two, try to let it go. After all, what's done is done.

> **Dr. Miriam Greene says:** Fetal alcohol syndrome is a concern if a woman consistently consumes large amounts of alcohol throughout the pregnancy.

Q. Is it safe to use a tanning bed while pregnant?

A. Exposure to sunlight and ultraviolet rays from tanning beds could be damaging to your skin, especially during pregnancy. The horror-mones of pregnancy may make your skin, like mine, much more sensitive and more likely to burn. You may also experience hyperpigmentation (dark spots), especially on your face.

This condition intensifies with exposure to sunlight and ultraviolet rays.

The freckles and spots that I developed on my face and hands became darker from the sun and never fully disappeared after pregnancy.

Dr. Miriam Greene says: There have been no studies done, thus far, that have proved tanning beds to be harmful to a developing fetus, but this type of UV exposure has not been proved safe during pregnancy, either. When in doubt, it's probably best to skip the tanning salon.

Q. Is self-tanner (in a bottle) safe for pregnant women?

A. I haven't been able to find any studies that show that self-tanners have any harmful effects on pregnant women or a developing fetus. I think it's because any chemicals they contain affect only the top layer of skin, which sheds frequently. Penetration of these chemicals into your bloodstream would be minimal.

Be aware that your skin might react differently to a self-tanner due to hormonal changes during pregnancy. You may develop a rash, have blotchy and uneven spots, or have the color of the tan turn out to be much different from what you expected. Applying a small amount to a hidden test area may be best to determine your skin's reaction.

46

Pregnancy Symptoms/Concerns

Q. I am suffering from bad edema and cannot remove my wedding ring. Is it safe to take *one* diuretic pill to allow me to get it off? I don't want to cut my ring if I can help it.

A. Most medications, including diuretics, are not recommended during pregnancy because of the possible risk to the fetus. Although taking just one may be okay, I recommend trying some natural alternatives before considering it.

Try getting your ring off during the time of day when you have the least swelling. For some women it's first thing in the morning. For others, it's right before bed. Before attempting the removal of your ring, try keeping your hand elevated above your head for an hour or so while lying down on your side. Then soak your hand in a dish of ice water for a few minutes. After your hand is slightly numb, dry it off and lubricate your finger well with dishwashing liquid or vegetable oil. If after several good yanks the ring does not come off, stop. The more you irritate your finger, the more it will swell. If this doesn't work, you may want to throw caffeine into this formula. Caffeine found in coffee, tea, and chocolate is a natural diuretic and may temporarily help reduce swelling. If this still doesn't work, you may want to visit your jeweler.

Dr. Miriam Greene says: 50 mg of vitamin B$_6$ (a natural diuretic) could help. As with any medications, check with your doctor beforehand.

Q. I'm five months pregnant and I have been craving bleach. I have a really strong urge to drink it. Can this be harmful to my baby?

A. Do not drink the bleach! It can be very harmful to you and your baby. You should report your craving to your doctor ASAP. You are probably deficient in iron or some other vitamin. Your body is instinctively seeking out what you are lacking through your seemingly odd craving.

It is more common than you think during pregnancy to crave such potentially poisonous items as permanent markers, spray paint, gasoline, dirt, and bleach. This is called a pica craving and is almost always an indicator of a dietary deficiency.

Q. I'm twenty-five weeks pregnant and am noticing an increase in fuzz on my face. Is it normal to grow facial hair during pregnancy? Will it go away?

A. The horror-mones of pregnancy can cause an increase in body and facial hair. This just "peachy" condition is quite normal, and thankfully the excess hair growth usually disappears shortly after childbirth.

Q. I used to have very curly hair. I'm on my third pregnancy and have noticed my hair getting straighter and straighter. Is this hormone-related? Will I ever have my curly hair back again?

A. It's possible that the horror-mones of pregnancy have changed your hair for good. My hair did just the opposite of yours. After each pregnancy, my thin, straight hair got thicker and wavier. The same thing happened to my sister.

Most people long for what they don't have (as far as hair types). I was happy with the change. If you really want your curly hair back, you may need to visit your local beauty parlor.

Q. I have been waking up at night feeling overheated and even breaking into a sweat. I dress lightly, put on the air, and even occasionally shower in the middle of the night to cool off. Is this normal, or is it a reason for concern?

A. It is natural for a woman's body temperature to be elevated during pregnancy. You are carrying around not only the extra pounds but also a little person that is a heat source on its own. Plus, the extra horror-mones of pregnancy can increase your body's circulation and temperature.

I remember that my body thermostat seemed to be most elevated in the evenings, during sleep. My husband used to be the one throwing off the covers in the middle of the night, leaving me shivering. When I was pregnant, the roles definitely reversed. I slept comfortably with nothing more than a sheet, while he required the sheet, two blankets, and a comforter. I also remember many nasty little fits of tugging and throwing of the linens. We finally had to resort to using separate covers to keep our amiable relationship intact.

> **Dr. Miriam Greene says:** Your basal metabolic rate goes up during pregnancy, and that causes a temperature rise.

Q. I am in my seventh month of pregnancy, and I notice that I am leaking colostrum from only one breast. Should I be concerned? Will I be able to breast-feed from only one breast?

A. I wouldn't worry. The breasts and milk glands develop, enlarge, and begin to produce colostrum, but not always at an equal rate.

I, too, had my left breast producing liquid many weeks before the right one caught up. By the time your baby arrives, I'm sure both of your boobs will be ready, willing, and able.

Q. Along with my morning sickness, I got what looked like hickeys all over my face and neck and had really red eyes from broken blood vessels. Is this from an iron deficiency or just some weird problem with my skin?

A. While vomiting from your morning sickness, many of your muscles, ligaments, and tendons constrict and put a major squeeze on blood vessels trapped in the area. Under enough pressure, these blood vessels will pop and show up as red splotches on the skin or red spots in the whites of your eyes. During pregnancy, your blood vessels are much more swollen and more prone to popping under pressure. Since you know the blood vessels in your face and neck are particularly sensitive, do remember to be careful while pushing during delivery.

Q. I have what seems to be a small skin tag on my vulva. I've heard about skin tags developing during pregnancy but assumed they would be under my arms or on my neck. Will it go away?! Can friction from intercourse cause skin tags?

A. It's true that the underarms and neck are usually the most populated by skin tags, but throw in the horror-mones of pregnancy and they can crop up just about anywhere. A friend of mine got one on her anus and assumed it was a teeny tiny hemorrhoid. Another friend got one on her nipple that she had to have removed, as it made breast-feeding very uncomfortable.

If your skin tag really bothers you, you can get it removed after the pregnancy. Intercourse will not cause skin tags around the genitals, but it may irritate them. You may want to make sure the tag is well lubricated so it doesn't get pulled and irritated during sex.

Dr. Miriam Greene says: Most skin tags that appear during pregnancy resolve in a few months after the pregnancy or, if breastfeeding, a few months after the baby is weaned.

Q. My mood swings are swinging all over the place. It has gotten so bad that my fiancé and I argue every day. What can I do to keep myself calm and my mouth shut?

A. Horror-monal hysteria, frequently experienced by pregnant women, is difficult to control at times. During pregnancy I found those biting, nasty comments flying out of me before I knew what I was saying. My mouth was acting faster than my brain, and it didn't take much to set me off.

Realizing that you are in the grip of pregnancy-induced hysteria is the first step to controlling it. The next time you feel yourself about to spit, "Shut up, you #@!-ing %#!@!!," try to take a moment and breathe. Attempt to remember what made you attracted to your fiancé in the first place. How did you fall in love? What was your first date like? If you can bring yourself to that pleasant place for just a moment, you may have a chance to break the spell of horror-monal hysteria and see things more clearly.

Q. I'm twenty-three weeks pregnant and have a cottonmouth with a very foul taste that doesn't change or go away with food or drink. I've tried drinking more water, brushing more, using mouthwash, and chewing gum. Nothing really works. Any idea what may be causing this?

A. The foul taste in your mouth is probably caused by your dry (cotton) mouth. Less saliva can cause certain stinky bacteria to become more active. Unfortunately, mouthwash, toothpaste, and gum don't do much to control these bacteria. Your best bet is to try keeping your mouth as moist as possible.

Drinking a lot of water helps. Also sucking on hard candies or lozenges can keep your mouth moist. The only drawback to candies is that most accelerate plaque growth and tooth decay, which can be more prevalent in pregnancy. Pregnant women have to be very conscientious about dental hygiene, so you should brush lightly several times a day.

Q. I am six weeks pregnant and suffering from terrible constipation. It has been thirteen days since I had a bowel movement, and nothing the doctor has suggested has worked. I am in pain and I already look like I am three months pregnant due to my distended belly. Help! I'm miserable. Any suggestions?

A. Constipation during pregnancy is due to the fact that a mother's body draws and retains more fluids for the growing baby, placenta, and amniotic fluid, therefore making the stool dry. You can try to conquer colon dehydration by drinking more liquids, but then you run the risk of increasing the already way too frequent urination problem.

I'm sure you've already tried all the usual remedies for constipation, such as eating plenty of fiber and drinking lots of water. One trick that worked for my sister is to drink two tablespoons of olive oil a day and then take a brisk walk.

Dr. Miriam Greene says: If you haven't had a bowel movement in over a week, you should notify your doctor. If constipation goes on too long you may have to be disimpacted.

Q. Whenever I manage to poop, I notice that my anus gets extremely swollen and looks as if it's actually been turned inside out. A flap of tissue pokes out of the anus opening and I have to push it back into me. Help! What's going on?

A. My term for your condition is "cauliflower butt," and yes, I've had it too. Cauliflower butt is brought on by building pressure, weight gain, and constipation, which in turn bring on hemorrhoids.

Hemorrhoids are almost unavoidable during pregnancy. Some women get them all throughout the pregnancy, while others develop them during labor and delivery.

There are two types of hemorrhoids—external and internal. An external hemorrhoid is a vein that pokes out through the muscle wall near the anus. It usually looks like a swollen blueberry or cherry sticking out. Poking it back inside your rectum may provide some temporary relief as less ballooning out of the vein means less discomfort. Internal hemorrhoids are the same thing, just inside of the rectum. This puffing out of veins around your rectum may give your butt a cauliflower appearance, thus explaining the term "cauliflower butt."

To help ease the swelling and pain of cauliflower butt, you might try an old trick of mine: After every bowel movement, gently clean the cauliflower with witch hazel pads (like Tucks) and then pack a bunch of clean pads on and around your anus. Change the pads every time you go to the bathroom. The witch hazel will cool the area and help reduce swelling.

Also, to keep your hemorrhoids from getting further aggravated, try not straining while having a bowel movement, keeping your feet elevated as much as possible, sleeping on your left side, using Preparation H and other topical medicines, and keeping bowel movements regular with stool softeners and/or fiber.

Dr. Miriam Greene says: Hemorrhoids are actually varicose veins in the hemorrhoidal veins.

Q. Sometimes I strain while trying to push out a BM. Can I hurt the baby if I push too hard? I keep having this (probably irrational) fear that I'm going to accidentally push the baby out, or cause some kind of permanent damage.

A. Straining while having a bowel movement will not harm the baby, but you could harm yourself in the end—and I mean your rear end. Constipation is a very common symptom of pregnancy, and so are hemorrhoids, which are often brought on by pushing too hard while pooping. Once you develop a hemorrhoid, this area of your rectum will be forever weaker and prone to future hemorrhoid episodes.

Being a Hemorrhoid Queen myself, I advise you to do all you can to stave them off, and if you do get them, do all you can to minimize them. Mine were so bad that I had to have surgery. I can honestly say it was the worst pain I've ever experienced—ten times more painful than a C-section, if you can believe that!

47

Sex, Orgasms, and Masturbation

Q. Is it safe to use a dildo while pregnant?

A. Barring any medical problems, dildo use is perfectly fine. If you are at a high risk for premature delivery, have problems with the placenta, experience unexplained bleeding, or your water has broken, you should abstain from intercourse—with a dildo or a live penis.

Q. Is it safe if I use a vibrator during my pregnancy? Will it cause *any* harm (hearing loss and so on) to the unborn child?

A. While it is true that by week five your baby's hearing ability is already developed, I don't think you need to be overly cautious about protecting your baby's hearing. After all, the uterus and amniotic fluid do provide somewhat of a buffer—similar to being underwater. If you were on a county road crew using a jackhammer on a daily basis, then you might have cause for concern.

If your vibrator is particularly loud, consider buying a quieter one or just using it on the outside for clitoral stimulation. Whatever you do, don't give up on masturbation. Orgasms during pregnancy can be the best of your life. Live it up!

Dr. Miriam Greene says: Vibrator use during pregnancy is okay, but I don't recommend inserting a vibrator into the vagina. As opposed to a penis that's attached to a body, a vibrator may penetrate too deeply and may possibly injure the cervix or induce labor.

Q. Is rough sex harmful to the baby?

A. If you are at high risk for premature delivery, have problems with the placenta, experience unexplained bleeding, or your water has broken, you should abstain from sex, and especially rough sex. Otherwise, I say go for it. With the exception of S&M or intercourse involving the insertion of sharp objects, the baby should be fine. The cervix, amniotic sac, and fluid provide the baby with a good barrier against big, jarring movements like rough sex.

Q. Is it safe to swallow sperm while pregnant?

A. You can safely ingest fluids or secretions from another human body as long as that body does not have some kind of communicable disease. I wouldn't recommend ingesting large quantities, though, as this may make you sick to your stomach.

Q. My husband says that sex with me hurts his penis, like he's running into a wall. I've never heard of anything like this. What is he talking about?

A. I suppose it is possible that your vaginal canal may seem shallower, especially if you are in the upright position, with the weight of your uterus pushing downward. In truth, though, your vaginal canal is actually expanding and becoming more elastic to eventually allow for the passage of the baby.

I suspect your husband's complaints are more psychological

than physical. Many men worry about bumping the baby with the heads of their penises during intercourse. This fear is bound to be distracting during the act, which could, in turn, make a man feel physically uncomfortable. Of course, sex will in no way harm or disturb the baby during a normal pregnancy. Talking about this with your husband may help. If he continues to complain of a hurt penis, you might try different positions, such as elevating your hips to pull the uterus away from his penis, or manual or oral sex.

Q. My fiancé thinks it's a turnoff to make love to a pregnant woman! He says he won't be able to look past the big belly and the baby inside me. Do you think he will change? Do other men feel this way? Am I really looking at several months of no sex? What can I do?

A. You'd be surprised how many men think this way. Some of them cannot get over the "Madonna complex" and view their pregnant wife as a mother, similar to their mother, which usually isn't a turn-on. Other men believe that sex with a pregnant woman may hurt the baby and they don't want to put their child at risk. Of course, this is ridiculous! And there are some men who are just not attracted to the physical aspects of a pregnant woman, such as the big belly, swollen vagina, and ballooning breasts. On the other end of the spectrum, there are also men who are even more turned on by the body of a pregnant woman.

Men's views on sex during pregnancy can stem from past relations with their mothers or what they were taught as a child, or may be based on one pivotal incident. Whatever the cause, I'm sorry to say there's nothing you can do to change your man's feelings. The only way he will change is if he thinks he should investigate and possibly work on his feelings. You might try suggesting this, but I don't advise forcing the issue.

In the meantime, if he doesn't come around, there's always your trusty vibrator! And don't worry, you will have your old body (maybe a little worse for the wear) back someday.

Q. I find many pregnant women to be incredibly sexy. Is that weird? I am a happily married father of three.

A. I see you are very in touch with your procreating instincts, which is perfectly normal. If men didn't find the female pregnant body attractive, most would stop after one child, don't you think?

Pregnant women also are sending a subliminal message to the male gender: "Pssst! Look at me, I've actually had S-E-X!"

Q. Is it normal not to desire sex at all during pregnancy? My husband has been great about it, but it's making me feel quite down. People keep telling me horror stories about lack of sex after the baby is born. Ours is due next week and I am afraid that this will go on forever. Am I alone?

A. I can assure you, you are not alone. Women's desire to have sex can vary drastically during pregnancy. Some women become complete horn dogs and want sex all the time, while others, like you, couldn't care less. There are a lot of factors that can contribute to your desire or lack thereof, such as discomfort, fatigue, and anxiety. It's true that right after the baby is born sex is almost impossible because of your body healing from childbirth, sleep deprivation, and hardly any time to yourselves. But who knows, maybe you'll have just the opposite problem. Maybe you'll physically crave sex so much more once the timing is right.

Q. I cannot stop thinking about sex and can't seem to get enough. Can masturbating every day or multiple times in a day hurt the baby?

A. It's completely normal to get all sexed up during pregnancy and want it more than ever. As with food cravings, I believe your body will tell you what you want and need during pregnancy. Barring any problems such as bleeding, severe cramping, placenta previa, or an incompetent cervix, masturbating several times a day should cause no worries. So go ahead and have that chocolate éclair and an extra orgasm for dessert!

Q. I've been having orgasms in my sleep and they've been so strong that they have woken me up. Although pleasurable, they are also painful, as I get bad cramps immediately afterward. Are these sleeping orgasms and waking cramps normal?

A. During pregnancy, elevated hormones can make orgasms much more abundant and easier to have. Pregnancy hormones can also induce vivid dreaming. The combination of the two will result in frequent "wet dreams," which are very normal (and quite enjoyable, I might add!) during pregnancy. And don't worry, uterine cramping immediately following an orgasm is completely normal too.

Q. Sometimes I experience bleeding after intercourse. When I'm on top and leaning forward, I don't bleed. Does the angle of penetration affect the cervix? What are the safest positions?

A. During pregnancy, the cervix becomes engorged with blood and very tender. It's no wonder that most pregnant women experience some bleeding during and after intercourse, which isn't harmful. To avoid bleeding, try sexual positions that don't involve deep, cervix-bashing penetration. Being on top gives you the most control of penetration depth. You can also try the missionary position, but push your legs downward and squeeze against your partner's hips to control depth.

Dr. Miriam Greene says: Report any kind of vaginal bleeding to your OB/GYN. There's a small possibility that bleeding could indicate a problem with the pregnancy.

Q. Will air bubbles in the vagina during sexual intercourse harm the fetus?

A. Only if air is blown or forced directly into a vagina without allowing it to escape—an air embolism could form, which could be harmful. Pockets of air that form in the vagina during intercourse can escape around the penis and/or when the penis is withdrawn. It can be pretty embarrassing, though. Vaginal farts can be completely uncontrollable and extremely noisy!

Q. I love making my wife's nipples leak during sex. She is five and a half months pregnant. Will this reduce the quality of the colostrum that our baby will need?

A. I don't think you need to worry about taking food out of your baby's mouth. Any colostrum that leaks or is expressed before the delivery should be considered a free sample. After all, what your wife is producing now isn't going to "keep" until the baby is born. After delivery, a mother's hormones turn on the switch for the major colostrum production that is meant for the baby. Immediately after delivery is when you may want to stop stimulating your wife's breasts, but she probably will be too tired to fool around anyway.

> **Dr. Miriam Greene says:** Warning: Breast stimulation during pregnancy may cause uterine contractions that could induce labor. You should stop nipple stimulation if your wife experiences any contractions and abstain from it for the duration of the pregnancy.

Q. I have placenta previa. My doctor told me not to have intercourse, but she did not say anything about having orgasms. Is it okay to have an orgasm when I have placenta previa?

A. If your doctor has advised against intercourse, it's probably because you may be at risk for premature labor or hemorrhaging if your cervix gets jostled. I hate to tell you, but I think this includes abstaining from orgasms as well. During orgasm, your uterus contracts and spasms, which may disturb your cervix. I hope you don't have long to go!

Q. I am six months pregnant, and when my husband and I have sex it takes me forever to have an orgasm. Is this normal? Sometimes I can't have one at all. But I want to have sex all the time and I get mad when he doesn't want to. Please help!

A. While some women experience the best sex of their lives while pregnant, others have difficulty. You may have trouble reaching orgasm because of subconscious inhibitions about your maternal body. Maybe it's difficult to get in a comfortable position that is most pleasurable for you. Or perhaps you are feeling rushed to have an orgasm because your husband doesn't seem to want sex as frequently as you do.

It's very common for pregnant women to become horn dogs and want sex all the time. Sometimes the husbands just can't keep up! The only way I ever "got enough" during pregnancy is when I supplemented my sex life with a vibrator. Try it. You might find that a vibrator fulfills your needs.

Q. I am seven and a half months pregnant. Some of my friends say that we should stop having sex after a certain time because it can hurt the baby. Is this true?

A. Most physicians and midwives today allow patients to have sex right up until the day of delivery, barring any medical problems.

Near the end of your pregnancy, you may find that sex can be even more pleasurable, as increasing pressure and blood flow to the vaginal area can make orgasms most intense.

It's believed that intercourse at the very end of a pregnancy may stimulate the softening of the cervix and the beginning of labor. This is a good thing, believe me. Take it from one who was ten days overdue!

If you are at high risk for premature delivery, have problems with the placenta, experience unexplained bleeding, or your water has broken, you should abstain from intercourse. Otherwise, go right ahead and have all the sex you want.

Q. I am six months pregnant and have been told by friends and family not to have oral sex performed on me. Is this true?

A. Barring any oral or genital diseases, oral sex performed on an expectant mother is perfectly fine. The only real differences from oral sex with a nonpregnant woman are the taste, smell, and appearance of the woman's vagina. The vaginal area will puff up in size and darken in color. The odor and taste of the vaginal fluids will also be different. Some partners are put off by this while others are even more turned on.

Q. At my last doctor's visit she said the head was down, engaged, and at zero station, but I am not yet dilated. Is it still safe to have sex with the head so low?

A. You can have intercourse right up until you go into labor or your water breaks, unless your doctor advises against it. It will in no way harm the baby for you to have sex with the head engaged, although it may be a little more uncomfortable for you, as the pressure of the dropped baby may make your cervix and pelvis much more sore and sensitive.

48

Vagina Issues

Q. My crotch area seems to be swelling at an alarming rate. It doesn't itch or burn. Could I have an infection?

A. A puffy, swelling vaginal area is quite normal. The progesterone your body is producing is turning up the volume on your sex organs, engorging them with blood and fluids. You may notice all of your mucous membranes (including the ones in your vagina) becoming much more lubricated and swollen as well.

My friend Grace and I fondly coined the term "cheeseburger crotch," as that's what it looked like she was stashing in her panties during pregnancy!

Q. My baby feels like she is trying to kick through my cervix and into my vagina. Is there any way she could dislodge my mucous plug or stimulate labor, or is this just normal?

A. Yes, it's annoying and painful at times, but quite normal. Your baby is probably sitting upright and you are feeling plenty of movement down below from the legs and feet. When she kicks directly at your cervix or bowels, you may suddenly suck in your breath with surprise or pain.

During my second pregnancy, I remember feeling a sharp pressure/pain deep within my vagina that most resembled the feeling one gets during a pap smear. I knew from experience that it must be the baby pushing or punching at my cervix.

I don't think you need to worry about your baby dislodging your mucous plug or stimulating labor. Your cervix should be pretty tightly sealed. It's meant to endure the trials and tribulations of the baby mambo.

> **Dr. Miriam Greene says:** Sharp and sudden pains could also be a sudden ligament pull, which is more common in a second pregnancy.

Q. I woke up in the middle of the night and found my underwear to be wet. I'm not sure if I urinated or what. I'm sixteen weeks pregnant.

A. It could just be vaginal discharge, which becomes increasingly abundant during pregnancy. The discharge may have accumulated in the vagina while you were lying down and then just spilled out into your underwear when you stood up. Sometimes this discharge can be thick and creamy, and sometimes it's thin and slimy.

Alternatively, you may be right. It could be urine. This stress incontinence can be common in early and late pregnancy. I lost track of how many times I wet myself during pregnancy.

Q. I am six months pregnant and have been getting yeast infections about every other week. Why is this?

A. Unfortunately, frequent yeast infections are very common during pregnancy, especially late pregnancy. The moisture, heat, and abundant blood supply in the vagina lay out the welcome mat for yeast infections.

In addition to any treatment your doctor may prescribe, try taking warm (not hot) baths twice a day while using a gentle, hypo-allergenic soap to wash; changing your underwear frequently as it becomes moist; wearing only loose-fitting, cotton panties; and when you can, don't wear underwear at all. Let your vagina get a good airing out.

> **Dr. Miriam Greene says:** A change of pH in the vagina during pregnancy can cause you to get yeast infections. If you have bad or frequent infections, ask your doctor for relief options.

Q. I heard that during pregnancy you shouldn't shave your vaginal area. Is this true and, if so, how does this harm anything during the pregnancy?

A. I've never had my doctor or anyone else advise against shaving, waxing, or trimming my vaginal area while pregnant. As a matter of fact, I think this is the time you'll need to "maintain the landscaping" the most. As the months progress, your "garden" will receive more and more viewing by doctors, nurses, and the like.

Do be careful in the later months while attempting to shave or trim yourself, though. At week thirty-seven of my second pregnancy I made an attempt at "maintaining the garden" by using my husband's electric razor. I hovered over the toilet and tried to shave by feel alone. I felt a little sting, brought the razor up from under my orb, and noticed a good amount of blood on the razor. I cut myself pretty badly. Needless to say, I did only a half-assed job on the trim.

Q. I sometimes feel like there are bubbles coming out of my vaginal lips. It freaks me out. Where is the air coming from? Is this normal?

A. Now that you mention it, I remember having that feeling, too. One of my girlfriends had her "bubbles" actually make noise. It's bad enough trying to explain uncontrollable gas during pregnancy, but to have vaginal farts as well? Oh, that's bad.

These vaginal bubbles form because, yes, air does get in there. During pregnancy, the vagina becomes more elastic and loose to accommodate the passing of a baby. You may not even notice, perhaps while bending down to pick up a pencil off the floor, that your vagina opens up a little bit and some air gets in. This air gets pushed out with movement or with the seemingly constant flow of vaginal discharge. Surprise, surprise!

Q. I'm only nine weeks pregnant and I've been having awful shooting pains in my crotch that come and go. Can you explain?

A. It sounds like the "stabbing vagina pains" I've experienced as well. It's quite embarrassing to have one of these pains suddenly strike in the presence of strangers. I once shook and gasped so loudly that everyone in line at the supermarket asked if I was okay. "Oh sure," I wanted to reply. "It's just a stabbing vagina pain."

I believe these are similar to the "stabbing uterine pains" and are caused by stretching and repositioning of tendons, ligaments, and muscles. Your innards have to rearrange themselves to make room for the baby, and sometimes this can cause abrupt pain.

Q. I am seven months pregnant and half of my outer vaginal area is swollen. I have had three other pregnancies and this has never happened. It feels like it is throbbing once in a while. There is no pain and it doesn't bother me. Do you know what is causing this?

A. Although I am no medical expert, I might guess at one of the following. Venal engorgement involves a vein popping through the muscle wall. As with hemorrhoids, you may feel a "throbbing" in the area. Uterine leiomyomas or fibroids are nonmalignant tumors that most commonly appear in the groin and can be aggravated during pregnancy and/or first materialize during pregnancy. Or, finally, it could be nothing.

In any case, you should consult your doctor ASAP, just in case.

Dr. Miriam Greene says: This is probably just a varicose vein in the vagina. If vaginal swelling becomes painful, you should contact your OB/GYN. Painful vaginal swelling could be a thrombosed vein or an inguinal hernia, which needs medical attention.

49

Miscellaneous

Q. How late into your pregnancy can you get a pedicure?

A. Until the doctor says it's time to push! Seriously, though, you can get a pedicure right up until the very end if you so desire. I was sure to have my toes done a few days before each of my due dates. Not only will your toes get a full viewing while being up in the stirrups, but also afterward when you have visitors in the hospital and your feet will most likely be propped up on the bed. Who wants to stare at long, gnarly, yellowing toenails?

Q. I just started a new job that I love and don't plan on leaving. I just found out that I am pregnant and I'm now worried about how to tell my boss. I'm also concerned about not being eligible for FMLA (the Family and Medical Leave Act). How should I handle this situation?

A. Since you are newly pregnant, you have plenty of time to tell your employer. You could even wait until you begin to show, which may not be for several months. At a minimum, I think you should at least wait until you are into the second trimester when it is statistically a "safer time." (I'm not saying that you will miscarry, but the odds of miscarriage are greater in the first trimester.)

If you work for a large company and are eligible for any type of health insurance, then you can request a copy of your insurance plan. This should include information and terms of maternity leave. If you have any questions, you can contact the health-care provider directly without your boss's knowledge.

If you work for a small business and do not have any type of health-care plan, then you may have to wait to broach the subject of the maternity leave.

When you do tell your employer, you should already have a clear idea of what you would like your plan to be after the baby is born. Are you going to continue working? How much maternity time would you like to have? Would you like to slowly return to the office environment, perhaps by starting part-time? Of course you may not get everything you request, but starting with an ideal plan is the best way to negotiate the process.

Q. My baby's heartbeat has always been extremely fast. At my latest appointment it was very slow. Is this normal, or something I should be concerned about?

A. If there was anything wrong with the rate of your baby's heartbeat, your OB/GYN would most likely notice and remark on it. In early pregnancy when the baby is very small, the heartbeat is faster. By the time the baby is born, the baby's heartbeat will have slowed considerably. Your baby's heart rate is probably slowing due to growth. Did you know that an elephant's heart beats at 35 beats per minute (bpm), while a mouse's heart rate is 600 bpm? A normal human fetal heart rate is between 110 and 160 bpm. Your baby's heart rate will differ depending on the age of the fetus and the activity level at the time.

Q. I'm twenty-eight weeks into my second pregnancy and the baby seems to be constantly moving. Is there any relation be-

tween a very active fetus and a cranky infant, or a less active fetus and a calm infant? I'm wondering if I have a baby crab in there.

A. As far as I can tell, there are no known studies on the subject of fetal movement relating to a child's disposition. I can tell you that with my first pregnancy, my baby was extremely active and she turned out to be a very calm, easy, and good-natured baby. During my second pregnancy, I think I had a normal amount of fetal movement. My second child turned out to be much more demanding, vocal, and moody. Regardless, I love them both the same.

Based on my experience, I don't think there's any way to predetermine the personality of your child. I guess you'll just have to wait and see!

Q. Although my husband and I are having the baby we planned for, we are fighting more and more. I know my hormones are raging, but it's like *he* is the one with too many hormones. I love him dearly and I know he loves me, but he's been so mean and acts as if everything about this pregnancy is inconveniencing him. I don't know how to handle it. MEN!!!!

A. Yes—men! They are so different from us. Their brains just don't function the same way. I cannot tell you how many times I've argued with my husband, trying to get him to see my logical point of view. Then I have to remind myself, Oh, yes, he is a man and does not think like me.

It sounds like your husband is going through the common new-father-to-be panic mode. He's probably playing through his mind again and again all of the changes and stresses this baby will bring to his life.

Most men usually do come around later on in the pregnancy. When your husband starts to see your rounding form, he may realize that little bun in the oven is actually his baby—a baby he'll be able to play with, teach, and have hopes and dreams for.

If your husband was similarly panicked before your wedding and was then surprised at how content he was with married life, I don't think you have anything to worry about. He is now just repeating his pattern—a common male pattern—and should improve his behavior soon enough.

Q. Any advice on how to handle a stressful pregnant wife? I seem to make my wife constantly irritated, she often blames me for only wanting to hurt her, and we have huge arguments daily. It is quite difficult for me to understand why she reacts so strongly to my "bad behavior." I am trying to find ways to calm her down, rather than putting "more wood on the fire."

A. The best way to handle a stressful pregnant wife is to really understand her. You need to know what's going on inside her body and mind. Actually being pregnant is the best way to relate, but since that's not possible for you, I'll try to give you an idea of what your wife may be feeling.

First, it's the horror-mones of pregnancy, which can make her mood swings so erratic and her temper extremely short. Believe me, you're not the only one subjected to her hostile behavior. I can remember in my last trimester of pregnancy feeling as if my nerves were constantly on the brink of the boiling point.

Second, your wife is experiencing a multitude of new and uncomfortable, if not painful, pregnancy symptoms on a regular basis. Pain and illness can make people bitter. It does take a toll on your tolerance and outward kindness toward others. I can remember thinking: If you are not experiencing back pain, Braxton Hicks contractions, heartburn, faintness, shortness of breath, nausea, fatigue, swollen legs, a sore pelvis, and throbbing feet, then you had better not give me any shit.

Third, you are the one who got her pregnant. I know this seems irrational, but if it weren't for you, she wouldn't be going through all of the discomfort and stress of pregnancy and childbirth. Is it really fair that the husband gets to drink wine with dinner, eat sushi, sleep through the night without heartburn, leg cramps, and Braxton Hicks, and still gets to become a parent to a sweet, tiny baby at the end of pregnancy?

Fourth, you are there. After time, everything and everyone become annoying during pregnancy. If your wife lived only with a dog for the duration of the pregnancy, the poor animal would spend many nights in the doghouse, so don't take it personally.

The good news is that your old wife is still in there somewhere and she will come back. You may even catch a glimpse of the old her every now and then after a bowl of chocolate ice cream or a really good orgasm. In the meantime, you may want to remember these few key phrases to get you through the rest of the pregnancy: Yes, honey. Right, honey. Anything you say, honey.

Q. **What are some things I can do to help myself begin to dilate? Is it true that semen from having sex can soften the cervix?**

A. Yes. It is true that semen can help facilitate labor by softening the cervix, although it never worked for me. I've found that labor started only when the baby was good and ready—it wasn't up to me at all. To encourage labor I tried taking long walks until my varicose veins were throbbing; swimming laps; frequent rough sex; and aerobic dancing. The aerobics and walking did bring on many bouts of Braxton Hicks contractions, but no labor.

At the end of the last trimester, most women are so uncomfortable and desperate for labor to begin they'll try anything. The above-mentioned tactics may or may not work for you. In the meantime, you can take a little time to pamper yourself while you still can. Get a pedicure, have your hair done, or put your feet up and catch up on some phone calls to friends and family before the baby arrives.

Dr. Miriam Greene says: If you are at term and have your doctor's permission, you might try raspberry leaf tea (can usually be found at health food stores) or castor oil to bring on labor.

50

Worries During Delivery

Q. How do I avoid any feces from coming out while pushing during delivery? It happened with the birth of my first child. The baby came out and so did some of my feces. It was *so embarrassing!*

A. Women with long labors usually do have one small advantage—diarrhea and plenty of time to empty out the bowels, while women with short labors sometimes find themselves pooping on the delivery table. Don't worry, most doctors and nurses have seen this many times before and are quite used to it.

The only thing I can think of to possibly avoid this situation is to give yourself a warm-water enema to clean out your bowels before heading off to the hospital. Or ask your attending nurse to give you one.

Twenty years ago it was common practice to give women enemas during labor. I suspect this no longer occurs today because women are more embarrassed to have the enema than to poop on the table!

Q. Do I have to shave my privates when I am pregnant?

A. There is no reason to shave during pregnancy unless you have a preference for it. As far as shaving for the birth, it used to be common practice for women's pubic hair to be shaved prior to delivering because doctors thought that eliminating the hair would decrease chances of infection. However, statistics showed that there were actually more instances of infection reported from shaving than not shaving. These days, the most common practice seems to involve swabbing the vaginal area in antiseptic before the birth.

Usually, the only time shaving is required is when you have a cesarean birth, as I did with my first child. They didn't shave very much, though—just a little off the top.

Q. I am six months pregnant, and I am an incredibly modest person. I was wondering if there's any way to remain at least slightly covered during my delivery? I am horrified at the thought of having everything out there for all to see, especially in front of my husband!

A. I, too, remember being quite concerned during my first pregnancy about the fact that many people were going to be staring at my crotch, possibly for hours, during the labor and delivery. I imagined being extremely humiliated and embarrassed. Well, I am happy to report that this did not happen and has never happened to anyone I know, no matter how modest she was. During labor in the hospital with all of the nurses and doctors examining you, modesty will be the farthest thing from your mind. Maybe labor releases some kind of anti-inhibition chemical. Or maybe it's the intensity of contractions that distracts you.

I know it seems hardly comforting now, but believe me that when the time comes, you won't care one little bit.

Dr. Miriam Greene says: I've had a few extremely modest patients who requested to have their bodies almost fully covered during labor. This kind of modesty usually lasts only through the early phase of labor. Once the active phase has begun and the contractions become more intense, they practically scream at me to remove that cumbersome drape.

51

Postpregnancy Issues

Q. I had my nipple pierced before I became pregnant. I have a hole on either side of my nipple, and when I squeeze it, a yellowish liquid comes out of the holes. It does not hurt. My biggest concern is breast-feeding. Will this interfere?

A. The yellowish liquid is colostrum, which is produced by the milk glands and is later replaced by real milk two to four days after the birth. Some women notice small amounts of colostrum leaking from their nipples before giving birth, but the bulk of it comes in after the delivery.

During pregnancy, you may notice little "buds" appearing on your nipples, which are milk ducts coming to a head. Did you know that milk can squirt out of each and every one of these ducts? There can be anywhere from twenty to fifty ducts in each nipple! I used to think the milk would neatly come out of one hole. Nope!

As far as having had your nipples pierced, I don't think you have anything to worry about. You may have severed a few milk ducts, but there are more than enough ducts to compensate and create a healthy milk flow.

Q. Is there a difference in a woman's hips spreading permanently postpartum if she delivers naturally versus by cesarean?

A. I think a permanent spreading or widening of the hips due to pregnancy depends on numerous factors. For example, if a cesarean section is performed before a woman goes into labor, the chances of the pelvis bone opening up are greatly decreased. Also, if your mother got wider hips after childbirth, then your chances for the same increase.

I had a cesarean section the first time because my pelvis didn't open up enough to allow the baby to pass. Afterward, I found my hips to be wider anyway. After my second childbirth experience, my pelvis did open and I succeeded in having a VBAC. My hips got wider still, as did my mother's when she gave birth. Ah, well, just chalk it up to another battle scar of pregnancy, I always say!

Q. Does this "cheeseburger crotch" go away?

A. Thankfully, yes, the cheeseburger crotch does go away. It normally takes a few weeks after delivery to have your vaginal area return to its former size. If you have a vaginal birth and/or an episiotomy or vaginal tears, it may take a little longer for the swelling to go down. Some women notice a looser vagina or longer labia, but many snap right back into shape. Vaginas are very elastic!

Q. I had my baby two months ago and I just got my period for the first time. Something the size of my pinky and looking like skin came out. I am freaked out! It was *not* a blood clot. Any ideas what it can be and if I should be concerned?

A. It was probably some leftover amniotic tissue or membranes that did not completely dispel until the full shedding of your uterine lining. I have come to find this is a lot more common in women who've had C-sections.

After the cesarean birth of my first, I had a large mass of tissue come out of my vagina after six weeks. I thought it looked like a Slim Jim! The grossest part was that it was still attached. I had to pull it out, and I felt a slight ripping somewhere inside. Yes, it was scary, and yes, it made me sick to my stomach! As it turns out, I was fine. I later learned it was some of the leftover amniotic sac.

Unless you notice a foul smell accompanying your vaginal expulsions or have unusual cramping or bleeding, you're probably okay. You should report this to your doctor on your next visit, though.

Q. I'm breast-feeding and now my breasts are not the same size. The right is small and the left is big and full of milk. Is this normal? Are my breasts ever going to be the same size again?

A. Don't worry; your lopsided boob problem is very common and quite normal. Sometimes the milk ducts in one breast are more active than the other. Sometimes the baby prefers to nurse more on one side than the other. In either case, you can end up with uneven breasts.

Usually, the larger breast is the one producing more milk. You would think that draining this breast would even out your proportions, but in fact, just the opposite is true. The more you have the baby nurse or try to pump the milk out of this breast, the more it grows and produces even more milk. And the less used breast begins to shrink and produce less. The trick is to try and nurse or pump more often on the smaller breast to make it catch up with the larger one.

Whether you get them to even out or not, it doesn't really matter. After you are done with breast-feeding, your breasts will both return to roughly the same size.

Q. I am flat chested—about an A-minus cup. Will this affect breast-feeding?

A. If you are pregnant, you won't be flat chested for long. During pregnancy, most women's breasts increase several cup sizes. Don't worry if your breasts still don't seem "big enough." It's not the size that provides an ample milk supply for the baby, it's the output of the milk ducts. For example, my huge-chested friend could usually pump only four ounces of milk at a time, while my much smaller boobs could produce twelve ounces in five minutes flat.

Q. Does breast-feeding cause sexual arousal? Or is it different with your baby?

A. During nursing and sex play, levels of the oxytocin hormone are increased. Oxytocin production peaks just before orgasm and it also triggers the "letdown" milk reflex for breast-feeding. Since this hormone is present in both scenarios, it's no wonder some women become aroused while breast-feeding. Although rare, some women may actually orgasm as a result. Don't worry if you feel aroused while breast-feeding. It's perfectly normal and does not mean you have pedophile tendencies.

Q. I am twenty-two years old and have two children, three and four years old. It seems my boobs just keep getting smaller. Why?

A. I, too, went through this very common (and normal) wilting breast dilemma. Before my first pregnancy I had perfectly perky 34C boobs. After, they were sagging sacks of 34As. I'm sorry to say most women's breasts do deflate a little bit more with each pregnancy. If you have a third child, they may remain the same or get even smaller still. The only times that I've ever known of someone's breasts actually getting bigger from pregnancy is when the pregnancy weight is not lost.

Aside from breast implants or getting pregnant again, the only thing you can do to improve your bust line is to buy yourself an extra-padded push-up bra. I, personally, found the Victoria's Secret Very Sexy or Miracle Bra collection to be the most realistic boob substitute.

Q. Since I've given birth I feel wide and loose in the vagina. My vaginal muscles never went back to the way they used to be. Is there something that can be done? Would it be covered by insurance?

A. It's more common than you think to have a looser vagina after giving birth. After all, it does stretch considerably to let a fully developed baby pass. Some women's vaginal skin and muscles tighten back up after birth, but never are quite as tight. Other women have real problems with too much looseness, like panty hose that never quite get their shape back. I think the elasticity of your vagina is mainly due to heredity.

If you plan to have more children, you should mention your discontent with the present state of your vagina. Some OB/GYNs will actually give you a few extra stitches while doing an episiotomy to correct a loose vagina. Or you can opt for having it surgically tightened now, but be sure you are done with childbearing. Most insurance companies cover the procedure if your OB/GYN agrees that your vagina needs corrective surgery.

Q. I've heard some women never get back to themselves, mentally, after pregnancy. A friend of mine used to keep such a nice house and care for herself, but during and after pregnancy she changed, and not for the better. Why does this happen to some women? Is there anything that can be done?

A. Depression is a common symptom of pregnancy and it may carry over into the first year or so after the baby is born—known as postpartum depression (PPD). Levels of these symptoms vary from woman to woman and even from pregnancy to pregnancy in the same woman. PPD is a very real and potentially damaging

symptom of pregnancy and postpregnancy and should not be ig-
nored. Unfortunately, some people don't take it seriously enough
and many women go untreated.

The first step is recognizing these symptoms and then making
a plan to do something about it. Visit www.postpartum.net and
www.postpartumNY.org for more detailed information.

Ultimately, you are the one in control of your body, your emotions, and your life. Being properly informed and aware of PPD
before the fact can be your biggest weapon against it.

> **Dr. Miriam Greene says:** Three to ten days after giving birth, post-
> partum blues (a general feeling of being down and weepy) can
> be normal. If the blues last for more than two weeks, and are ac-
> companied by extreme downs of depression, anger, or feelings
> of harming the baby, you should consult your doctor immediately.

Q. I had a baby two months ago and my skin pigmentation in
some areas (genitals, armpits, and anal area) is still darker than
usual. Will this ever fade? What can I do? Will it get darker if I
tan?

A. You still have some time for your dark-skinned areas to fade.
Sometimes it takes a few weeks, sometimes several months. But
do be aware that in most cases the skin on your nipples, genitals,
and anal area will be darker forever. Maybe not as dark as during
the pregnancy, but they probably won't revert back to the color
they once were.

As for these areas getting darker if you tan, I doubt it, unless
you tan naked, arms up to the sun, and spread-eagle.

> **Dr. Miriam Greene says:** Hyperpigmentation caused by pregnancy
> usually fades considerably about four months after delivery or
> four months after breast-feeding.

Q. I had a baby three weeks ago via C-section and have been told not to have vaginal intercourse for several weeks. Is there any reason I should not have anal intercourse now? I cannot find *any* information anywhere.

A. You probably cannot find any information on the subject because no medical professional would condone the act of anal intercourse. The reasons for this are loosely based on health issues and politics. Did you know that anal sex is still considered a crime in many states? I think that's ridiculous.

Okay, back to the issue here. You can probably resume anal intercourse as long as you get an okay from your OB/GYN first. When you are given the green light, do be careful not to be too rough. The tissue inside and surrounding the anus may be delicate and prone to tearing, as it could still be puffy with postpregnancy swelling. Slamming or jarring movements may also put your cesarean scar at risk for rupturing.

> **Dr. Miriam Greene says:** I advise my patients not to have intercourse of any kind—vaginal or anal—for eight weeks after a cesarean section to avoid infections.

Q. I had a C-section about four weeks ago and my uterus doesn't seem to have gone down much. I look like I'm five months pregnant. How do I get rid of my belly?

A. Don't worry. You're completely normal. No one ever goes home from the hospital without a still-pregnant-looking belly. I remember about six weeks after I had given birth, my Aunt Nancy came for a visit. The first thing she said to me was, "You're still fat!" I wanted to retort, "Oh, yeah? Well, so are you and you didn't even have a baby!" but I held my tongue. It takes several weeks, if not months, for the uterus to heal and return to its former shape and size.

Since you've had a C-section, it will take a little longer for you to heal and to be able to do some rigorous strengthening exercises, such as sit-ups and crunches. You can start by doing some walking and some slow crunches and gradually build yourself up to an exercise regimen. The bottom line is, give yourself a break. You've just had a baby and that's very hard work in itself!

Index

"dropping of baby," 139, 144
   sexual intercourse after, 207
drugs. *See* medications

ears, popping or clogged, 10, 104
eating too much, 92–93
   and diarrhea, 43
edema. *See* swelling
effacement, 139
embolism, in vagina, 205
emotions
   aggressive, during pregnancy, 73
   about being overdue, 151–52
   intense and volatile, 12, 16–18,
      101, 102–3
   negative, during pregnancy, 66
   toward marital partner during
      pregnancy, 66, 67, 69, 72–73,
      108–9, 215–17
   See also depression; moodiness
enemas, during labor, 219
engorgement, of vagina, 9, 82, 84,
   208, 211–12, 223
epidural block, 128, 129, 164–65
episiotomy, 130, 168
exercise, 22–23, 38–39
   and back pain, 83
   questions regarding, 185–87
extremities, swelling of, 9, 15,
   123–24, 148
eyes, red, 195

facial blemishes
   from vomiting, 195
   See also skin
facial hair, increase in, during
   pregnancy, 193

faintness, 10, 26, 143, 148, 151. *See
   also* breathing
falling in love with baby, 116–17,
   170, 172
falls, 93–94
false labor. *See* labor
Family and Medical Leave Act
   (FMLA), 213
farts, 72–73
   vaginal, 205, 210–11
fast food, 46
fat, being mistaken for, when
   pregnant, 45
fatigue, 10, 28, 34, 85, 86, 126, 143,
   148, 151, 189
   after birth, 172
feces, coming out during delivery,
   219
feelings. *See* emotions
fetal alcohol syndrome, 190
fetal monitors, 130
fetal movement, and child's
   disposition, 214–15
fetal stress test, 159
fetus
   acoustic stimulator for, 178–79
   active time of, 178–79
   "dropping" of, 139, 144, 207
   heartbeat, 27, 214
   hiccups of, 10–11, 113
   listening to, on Doppler monitor,
      52, 62
   movements of, 7, 61–62, 71, 72,
      73, 83, 99, 113, 178–79, 208–9,
      214–15
   questions regarding harm to,
      188–91

About the Author
and Medical Contributor

Stacy Quarty

Stacy Quarty is a mom and graphic designer living and working in Southampton, New York. She came up with the idea for her book shortly after 9/11, when her graphic-design career took a nosedive. At home with a two-year-old and newly pregnant, Quarty, who had always wanted to write a book, realized that the ideal topic was right under her nose.

Quarty also hosts a weekly bulletin board on FranklyPregnant .com. The site gets more than 150,000 hits a day, has more than 1,000 pregnancy Q&As archived, and still continues to grow like an expanding maternal belly.

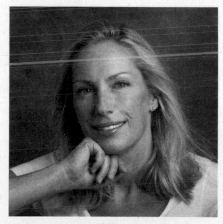

Quarty joined the Herstory writing group shortly after beginning her manuscript. While honing her writing skills, she became a leader in the development of the group. Quarty designs and donates all printed promotional materials for Herstory and also designs and maintains the Web site, www.herstorywriters.org. She chaired the Herstory annual benefit in 2003.

Stacy Quarty graduated from Long Island University with a B.F.A. in fine arts and an M.A. in graphic design in 1989. She minored in English literature and journalism.

Miriam Greene, M.D.

Dr. Miriam Greene practices obstetrics and gynecology in Manhattan and is an assistant professor at New York University School of Medicine. An interest in women's health developed early in Dr. Greene's medical school career and has remained a focus ever since.

In addition to her private practice, Dr. Greene has contributed her expertise in multiple print and broadcast media. Dr. Greene served as a medical consultant and actress on HBO's *Sex and the City*, is a medical adviser (OB/GYN) to *Family Circle* magazine, contributed a foreword to Janis Graham's *Your Pregnancy Companion* (Pocket Books, 1991), and has been interviewed and quoted by *Shape* magazine (spring 1995), *Newwoman* magazine (May 1995), the Associated Press (1997, 1998), and *Family Circle* (multiple contributions).

Dr. Greene has also been keynote speaker for Women's Health Awareness (December 1998) and featured guest on National Public Radio (August 1999).